The Cortical Monkey and Healing

Diagnosis

Prognosis

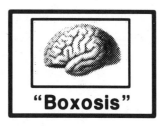

"Boxosis"

The brain boxed-up in the boxes

Majid Ali, M.D.

Library of Congress Cataloging-in-publication Data

Ali, Majid
The Cortical Monkey and Healing \ Majid Ali.--Ist ed.

Includes bibliographical references
1. Molecular medicine 2. Preventive medicine
3. Psychosomatic medicine 4. Somatopsychic medicine
5. Self-regulation 6. Auto-regulation
7. Healing

TXu 419-654   1990   ISBN 1-879131-00-5
10 9 8 7 6 5 4 3 2 1

Published in the U.S.A. by

Institute of Preventive Medicine
320-Belleville Ave
Bloomfield, New Jersey,07003
(201) 743-1151

Dedication

*This book
is dedicated to my
patients whose conquest
of their chronic diseases
without drugs gave me unequivocal
evidence that self-regulation works,
and that it must be accepted and advanced
as a medical discipline with predictable clinical
results.*

The case histories included in this volume, and the two companion volumes *The Pheasant and Suffering in Illness* and *The Dog and the Dis-ease Syndrome*, are true to life. Names and genders have been changed to protect the identity of the subjects.

Psychosomatic and somatopsychic models of disease are artifacts of our thinking.

Diseases are burdens on biology. These burdens are imposed upon our genetic make-up by our external and internal environments. The intensity of suffering caused by these burdens is profoundly influenced by a third element: the choices we make in our response to these burdens.

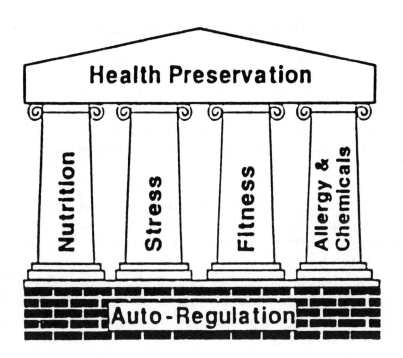

An expression of gratitude

For this book and my work in self-regulation which led to it, I am deeply grateful to all my teachers and friends. It is not possible to name all of them. Still, I wish to recognize some of them.

First, there are my teachers and friends who wrote the books which I have read over the years. Spoken word, on occasion, has sent me a flash of insight, but it is the written word which has given me that " body of water one swims in". These teachers include scribes of antiquity, philosophers of the classical times, observers of Nature of the medieval times, thinkers of the Age of Reason and the researchers of modern times.

Second, there are my teachers and friends at Columbia University, the American Academy of Environmental Medicine, the American Academy of Otolaryngic Allergy, the American College of Advancement in Medicine and the Meninger Clinic. I have had the high privilege of ready access to some of the most gifted researchers and astute clinicians in the fields of academic pathology, immunology, allergy, human ecology, and self-regulation.

Third, there are my teachers and friends at Holy Name Hospital, Teaneck, New Jersey. Sometimes I wonder if I have a " squint " of the mind. That might explain the pull for me of the *improbable*. Caring for the sick is a heavy responsibility. In clinical medicine, one must resolve the problems of the present as one engages the possibilities of the future. My colleagues at Holy Name saw to it that our patients were not hurt by my work with *auto-regulation*. I have been blessed with a very large number of friends at Holy Name, too numerous to be named here. Evalynne Braun, M.D. and Verna Atkins, M.D., my associates in the Department of Pathology and Alfred Fayemi, M.D., who was my associate for ten years, made special contributions to this book. Sister Patricia Lynch, President of the hospital, has been supportive of my work with self-regulation and environmental medicine. For this I must express my deep gratitude.

Fourth, there are my patients (and teachers) at the Institute of Preventive Medicine, Bloomfield, New Jersey to whom I dedicate this book.

Fifth, my dearest friend, Talat. She has been my teacher and constant companion. In some months, we will have been married for 25 years.

Contents

Preface

This book is about choice

In chronic illness we have a choice.

We can accept a chronic illness as a disease to be treated with a specific "drug of choice" and, in essence, suppress the symptoms.

Or,

We can look at a chronic illness as a burden on our biology. We can try to recognize this burden and understand how it causes illness. We can become sensitive to our biology, be responsive to it, and learn to regulate it. We can self-regulate and heal. This book is about this choice.

This book is about a changing medicine for a changing time

This is a time of a profound change in medicine. It is a time of an important discovery: that the dominant chronic problems of our time can no longer be treated with drugs.

There is a new possibility of a *Molecular Medicine*. It is the practice of medicine based on what the molecules *can* do to reverse disease rather than on what they *did* do to cause it. This medicine has four faces: Nutritional Medicine, Environmental Medicine, Medicine of Self-regulation, and a Medicine of Fitness. What binds these four disciplines together is molecular pathology. Cellular pathology gives us windows to injured tissues and cells *after* the injury has occurred. Molecular pathology gives us insights into the molecular and electro-magnetic events which initiate cell injury *before* the cells have been damaged.

Rudolph Virchow, the father of modern pathology, published *Cellular Pathology* in 1858 and liberated us from the restrictive tenets of gross pathology of medieval and ancient times. Now molecular pathology must liberate us from the restrictive tenets of cellular pathology in areas where cellular changes do not tell us how the disease begins.

New knowledge is defining new directions. Acute illness will remain a preserve of safe surgery and potent drugs; chronic illness, by contrast, is becoming a province for self-regulation. This time will be remembered as a time when self-regulation and healing moved from the fields of mysticism to the domains of science. It will be remembered as a time when the physician was displaced from the center stage in the arena of health and disease and the patient cast as the principal player. It was a time when the physician became a tutor and the patient a pupil.

Most chronic diseases of our time arise from problems of nutrition, stress, fitness, allergy and sensitivity to chemicals. Susceptibility to recurring viral and other infections usually occurs when a person's immunity has been damaged by these factors. Drugs are not an acceptable answer to these problems.

This book is about healing energy

Life is created with energy. Life is sustained with energy. Life ends when energy is depleted. When injured, molecules, cells, tissues and organs heal with energy. It stands to reason that the subject of healing cannot be separated from the subject of energy.

Why was it that the words "healing" and "energy" carried heretical connotations in medical circles? It is not a difficult question to answer. Medicine is a branch of science. Science is measurements and reproducibility. Historically, energy could not be measured in the context of healing. What could not be measured, women and men of medicine reasoned, was not worth scientific inquiry.

Now that healing energy can be measured with modern technology, should the "healing energy" be restored to its rightful place in clinical medicine? Patients speaking out in this book give eloquent answers to this question.

This book is about lessons learned from patients

Clinical history has always been regarded as the bedrock of

clinical medicine. So it ought to be.

When does the history fail a physician? This does not happen because the patient has nothing to say. He always does. Nor does it happen because the physician does not want to know what ails his patient. Contrary to some opinions, he always does.

History fails the physician every day in this age. It happens when the patient knows what he has to say is contrary to the prevailing medical dogma. He does not wish to challenge the knowledge of the physician and risk offending him. So he does not say what he needs to say. The physician does not hear what he needs to hear. History fails the physician. The patient pays for it. The price often is exorbitant.

This book is about kindness

Biology teaches us how to be kind to our body tissues. Anger and hostility are the first casualties of self-regulation. Biology, unburdened and set free, restores a person to a natural state of a kind awareness of his body tissues. Good health follows as a consequence. Kindness to others flows spontaneously and effortlessly from kindness within.

This book is about being kind to our body organs, tissues, cells and molecules.

Biology is the greatest of all teachers

Our biology never lies to us nor does it ever accept lies from us. People often question the judgement of their physicians. People in the throes of chronic illness are often uncertain about their own judgement. Patients do not question the workings of their own hearts, arteries, muscles, brain, blood stream, and other organs when they see them on video and computer screens, or in appropriate electro-magnetic fields. These signals from biology are unmistakable and irrefutable.

In this book, my patients speak about insights in biology which led them to elements of self-discovery at a "biologic-intuitive" level. What begins innocently as a method for control of migraine, asthma, or arthritis eventually leads to higher states of awareness of the human condition.

Psychosomatic and somatopsychic models of disease are artifacts of our thinking

Diseases are burdens on biology. Human intellect and human body organs are integral parts of the human condition. To separate them, as Socrates lamented, is to negate the completeness of the human condition.

Our technology has rendered irrelevant the debate of psychosomatic and somatopsychic nature of diseases. Advances in behavioral biology and experimental psychology have put these two disciplines on a collision course; a complete merger between the two is simply a matter of time.

Hope is a molecular event. So is dejection. Neuropeptide research is closing in on defining emotions and behavior as chemical sequences. Teilhard de Chardin dreamed of the day when man's technology would have conquered oceans and winds and would begin to explore the energy of love. We are seeing the dawn of that day.

Self-regulatory methods bring about profound changes in human biology. I describe in various sections of this book biochemical, electo-magnetic, and high-resolution microscopic changes that I have observed with *auto-regulation* in my patients. Clinically, most of my patients can control asthma and arthritis, lower blood pressure in hypertension, and normalize overactive and underactive thyroid glands with consistency and predictability.

It is unusual for me to see a patient who is unable to learn how to alter one or more electro-physiologic responses during his very first training session with me in our *auto-regulation* laboratory.

A surgeon's scalpel never heals. An internist's drug never heals. Organs, tissues, and molecules have an innate ability to heal. What the scalpel and the drug do is to remove impediments in the way of healing. *Auto-regulation* works exactly the same way.

Words are codes for images

For a physician, the name of a disease is a word which carries some images of healing. These are images of diagnosis, treatment, and prognosis.

For a patient, the name of a disease is a word which carries images of pain, suffering, disability and, sometimes, death. It does not carry any images of healing. But, what if this were changed. What if the name of the disease carried clear images of healing for the patient? Could the patient then heal himself? Patients in this book give clear and resounding answers to this question.

The name of a disease (diagnosis) sets the patient up, either for disease reversal with self-regulation, or for chemical dependence on drugs. This is a crucial distinction.

Different burdens on biology cause different diseases. Different diseases afflict us in different ways. Different afflictions require different corrective approaches, and different time-frames. Patients understand this well. None of this invalidates the basic principles of *auto-regulation.*

Medical statistics are of little relevance
to an individual patient.

In the prevailing dogma of the 3 Ds (a single disease, a single diagnosis, and a single drug of choice), medical statistics are established by a double-blind cross-over model of investigation. In this research design, both the patient and his physician are blinded to the nature of the treatment used so that they cannot in any way influence the results. It systematically strips the patient of all control over his treatment. By definition, it excludes from the final outcome any role that a patient may play in his own recovery, whether it is in areas of nutrition and fitness or in self-regulation.

The validity of the double-blind cross-over model is obvious when it is used for short periods of time for acute diseases and potent (and toxic) drugs. For chronic disorders, it creates spurious data. First, I know from personal experience that no physician or patient can truly be blinded about the nature of the treatment being used for any significant length of time (I assume that both have some measure of curiosity). Second, few patients will mindlessly follow *only* what their physicians prescribe while they suffer from a chronic illness. Nutritional, physical, and self-regulatory changes are invariably made by patients *to varying degrees.* There are still other important issues about accepting this *blessed* double-blind cross-over model as the gold standard in the treatment of chronic disease.

The critical issue here is that a patient must not allow anyone to set limits upon his ability to self-regulate and heal based on any medical statistics.

Absence of disease is not always presence of health.

With some exceptions, established diseases are not sudden departures from health. Diseases of our times are burdens on biology and immune dysfunctions caused by the problems of stress, poor nutrition, sensitivity to environmental pollutants, allergy, fitness, and susceptibility to viruses, bacteria, and other microbes.

Stress is an integral part of our biology. It is an ever-changing, kaleidoscopic mosaic of reticulated molecular events. Stress and anaphylaxis, it seems, belong more to Chaos physics (the new physics of turbulence) rather than the established Newtonian model. Nature designed the stress response for a survival advantage. Nature also gave us built-in mechanisms to switch off this reaction when it has served its purpose. The dominant health problem of our time is this: life in our time is an unrelenting stress. Before we can turn off the stress reaction to one stressor, we are confronted with another.

Drugs are not acceptable long-term substitutes for Nature's own molecular balancing acts. Drugs only suppress symptoms and postpone the inevitable tissue injury inflicted by unrelenting stress.

Our nutrition is in double jeopardy. Our food is often depleted of nutrients. Each meal challenges our biology with pesticides, insecticides, and antibiotics. Tissue damage caused by these elements is slow to appear, but cumulative.

Drugs dull our sensitivity to subtle, but progressive impairment caused by problems of nutrition.

In synthetic chemicals, we have unleashed a monster. The statistics for global environmental pollution are staggering. The incidence of illness caused by these agents (the Environmental Illness Syndrome) is rising at an alarming rate, and so is the occurrence of the classical hayfever type of allergy.

Drugs compound the problems caused by environmental illness and allergy.

Life in our time is robbing us of spontaneity in our physical activities. The recent trends and emphasis on fitness are promising. Still, I see many athletically oriented young women and men who suffer from chronic fatigue. I do not think that athletics alone can spare us from the hazards of modern living. Drugs are not acceptable remedies for energy and vitality.

Diseases are not drug deficiency syndromes

The true answer to our health problems is in knowledge. American society recognizes that our illnesses are not chemical deficiency syndromes to be healed by supplying the missing chemical as a drug. It is self-evident. The issue is not that people do not see this and do not want self-regulation. The issue is that they generally do not have access to professionals who are willing and able to provide the necessary insights and support, with care, compassion, and persistence. I am an optimist. I believe it will happen. In the future, patients will have access to such professionals.

"It is too simple"

Ken Gerdes, M.D. of Denver, an internist and a close friend, was among the group of physicians who attended my first *auto-regulation* workshop for physicians. He wrote a letter to me on his way back to Denver. He thought my discussion of the molecular basis of aging, accelerated aging, potential for intervention, and treatment of disease with *auto-regulation* was rational, logical, and scientifically sound. Further, he had no difficulty accepting the clinical results I was seeing with my *auto-regulation* methods. "I have been thinking about it all day," he wrote. "I am troubled about one thing though. It is too simple."

During the first two years of my work with *auto-regulation*, I was also troubled, sometimes deeply troubled, about the utter simplicity of the principles and practice of *auto-regulation*. As I closely observed more and more of my patients resolve their various chronic diseases without drugs, I recognized I had to make a choice:

*I could dismiss as apocryphal the accounts of
my patients (consider them innocent, or worse,
deceitful) and stop my work in self-regulation.*

Or,

*I could accept self-regulation as a valid medical
discipline which gives us predictable clinical
results, and continue my work to advance this
field.*

I chose the second option.

After I gave my very first *auto-regulation* workshop for
physicians, three of 14 physicians from this group incorporated
auto-regulation in their clinical practice. Since then, after each
workshop I receive calls from physicians affirming one or more
aspects of *auto-regulation* in the clinical practice of medicine.

This ongoing peer review has been most valuable to me. It
has sustained me during many periods of self-doubt and
discouragement.

When a person attends to a part of his biology, it responds.

This is the core idea of *auto-regulation*. It appears to be a simplistic and an improbable notion. How can the simple notion of attending to a body part elicit a response from it? How can such a response bring about a healing effect? How can "real" diseases be just wished away? How can the "hard science" of biology succumb to such a "soft" notion? Is it plainly not a case of some delusive possibility? I know how some people would answer these questions. My own response to these questions would have been simple disbelief during my over 30 years of study and practice of medicine. That was before I started my work with *auto-regulation*.

I would gladly accept all this. The problem for me has been this: this simple and improbable idea, and the *auto-regulation* methods based on it, have worked for most of my patients, not on an "anecdotal" or an "exceptional patient" basis, but in a consistent and predictable fashion.

This book is about this idea.

Majid Ali, M.D.

Teaneck, New Jersey.
July 4, 1990

Auto-reg and Molecular Medicine

The terms *"auto-reg"*, *"auto-regulation"* and *"Molecular Medicine"* appear throughout this book. This is a short note about these terms.

In my early clinical work, I set out to do some "stress management" for some patients with chronic indolent problems which seemed refractory to the standard prevailing medical methods. I found myself teaching these patients how to slow their hearts, open their arteries, and dissolve their muscle tension. In medical terminology, these activities are referred to as autonomic functions. It seemed logical to use the term "autonomic regulation" for it. My patients abbreviated this to *"auto-reg"*.

I soon realized my patients needed, and wanted, me to teach them methods for self-regulation and healing. I also recognized that self-regulation goes far beyond any ideas of autonomic regulation. I started a search for a simple term which, in practical terms, would declare our purpose.

Again, my patients solved my problem. They stayed with the term *auto-reg* as I experimented with different words. In the end I decided to follow their lead.

Looking back, my work with *auto-regulation* evolved in the

following sequence.

* *Stress management*

* *Autonomic regulation*

* *Self-regulation and healing*

* *States of consciousness*

One of the essential lessons my patients taught me is this: slowing the heart rate, keeping the arteries open, and slow, even breathing profoundly affect our mood and state of the mind. These basic methods of *auto-regulation* are very effective in dissipating anger and anxiety even when that is not our intended purpose. But this is just a beginning. *Auto-regulation* reveals the path of self-regulation and healing. A passage through the realms of self-regulation inevitably ushers a person to the higher states of awareness and consciousness.

Auto-regulation
is self-regulation and healing with energy.

Auto-regulation, as defined in this volume, is self-regulation and healing with energy, energy of tissues, cells and molecules.

It is self-regulation with full benefits of the science and technology of modern medicine. It is self-regulation with objective, measurable, and reproducible electro-magnetic, molecular, and cellular changes in our biology.

Auto-regulation
is not healing with counselling,
analysis, regression, hypnosis, or biofeedback.

****

A "body-over-mind" approach to healing

We often hear about the concept of healing with mind-over-body approach. In my own work with self-regulation, I do not find this to be sufficient for reversing chronic indolent diseases. I see superior clinical results when my patients adopt a *body-over-mind* approach, i.e. when they learn how to listen and attend to their tissues, and shut out their thinking minds.

We take pride in our minds, but healing is not an intellectual function. Healing cannot be forced upon injured cells and tissues by a demanding mind. Rather, healing occurs when the tissues are set free from the ceaseless censor of the mind. My patients were unable to control their asthma and migraine attacks, lower their raised blood pressure, or reverse other chronic illnesses with a *mind-over-body* approach.

In my own clinical work, a *body-over-mind* approach has given me far superior results. Many of my patients reversed their tissue injury and chronic diseases when they learned how to *attend* to their tissues. Tissues evidently know how to respond. We need only to learn how to shut our thinking *cortical* minds and attend *limbically* to our molecules, cells, and tissues in duress. This is not simply a clever play on words. Molecular repair and healing are visceral and *limbic* functions. Molecules, cells and tissues do respond when we attend to them.

Molecular Medicine

I use the term Molecular Medicine to refer to a practice of medicine based on molecular events which occur *before* cells and tissues are injured by the disease. Molecular Medicine is not based upon what we observe in cells with the microscope *after* the cells have been damaged.

In Molecular Medicine, treatment protocols are formulated

based upon the knowledge of the structure and function of molecules and the molecular requirements of the patient; the "science" of outcome studies substantiates the validity of these protocols.

Living things are composed of two families of molecules: the "oxidative aging molecules - OAMs" which are there to make certain that no life-form lives for ever; and "life span molecules - LSMs" which are there to make sure that living things do get a chance to live their expected life spans. The balance between OAMs and LSMs, in essence, is the basic equation of life.

Health, in molecular terms, is the molecular mosaic which balances the LSMs against the OAMs; disease, a state of molecular disarray in which the OAMs overwhelm the LSMs.

How do we reverse the molecular disarray which is disease? How do we restore the molecular mosaic which is health? By replenishing the LSMs and by excluding or holding in abeyance the OAMs. The former can be generated with protocols of Nutritional Medicine and of Medicine of Fitness; the latter can be excluded by the protocols of Environmental Medicine and those of the Medicine of Self-regulation. What binds these four disciplines together is the common thread of molecular dynamics. The clinical application of these molecular dynamics to treatment of disease is the practice of Molecular Medicine.

Section 1

A Tale
of
Two Stone Walls

A Blind Man's Stone Wall

A blind man touched a stone wall and leaned against it.

" This is the boundary of the world," he said.

A proverb

Dhobidharma's Stone Wall

Dhobidharma, an ancient sage, often travelled to different lands. His reputation preceded him wherever he went. On one occasion, Dhobi travelled to a kingdom. The king had heard of Dhobi and was thrilled with the possibility of meeting him. He ordered festivities on a grand scale to welcome Dhobi.

On the day of Dhobi's arrival, the king led his courtiers in a welcome party. A short distance out of the city, the king saw Dhobi standing still, intently gazing at a low stone wall. In reverence, the king stopped at a distance and looked at Dhobi. Dhobi did not move. Time passed by. The courtiers became tired and restless. Finally, the king spoke up,

" What were you looking at, your honor?"
" A stone wall," replied Dhobi.
" What do you see, your honor? "
" A wall no more," answered Dhobi.

In a chronic illness, we have a choice.

We can look at our skin as the blind man looked at his stone wall. We can relinquish charge of our biology, look to drugs for temporary suppression of symptoms,and accept the long-term consequences of chemical damage to our tissues.

Or, we can look at our skin as Dhobi looked at his wall. We can learn to dissolve it and see what is hidden beneath it.

We can move the "boundary".
We can see beyond the "wall".

We can become sensitive to our biology, be responsive to it, and learn to regulate it. We can recognize the dis-ease state and disease as a biology under different burdens and stresses. We can learn methods for removing these burdens and dissipating these stresses.

We can acquire self-regulatory skills for dissolving pain and suffering caused by the disease. We can self-heal.

Treating a disease is not the same
thing as caring for a person.

During the last twenty five years, I have had the opportunity to perform pathologic examination of over 75,000 biopsies and surgical specimens. During the same period, I directed a laboratory which performed more than fifteen million blood and other diagnostic tests. In clinical practice of medicine, I have had the opportunity to treat a fairly large number of patients in the fields of surgery, emergency medicine, allergy, immunology, ecology, nutrition and self-regulation.

I have sometimes thought about what my answer would be if I were asked to identify the principal failure of modern medicine. I will unhesitatingly say it is our failure to see the difference between *caring* for a patient and *treating* his disease. It is our failure to look at the electro-magnetic and molecular events which initiate disease. It is our failure to see the names of most chronic disorders as mere diagnostic labels. Caring for an ill patient calls for recognition of all the burdens on his biology; treatment of disease, as we are brought up to believe, is a simple matter of choosing *the drug of choice.*

"You treat asthma?"
"No, I don't."
"No?"
"No."
"But I thought you had a special interest in asthma."
"Yes, I do."
"And you don't treat asthma?"
"No, I don't."
"I listened to a tape of your lecture at the Academy meeting. You describe excellent results for patients with asthma."
"Yes, I did."
"If you don't treat asthma, where do you get your numbers from?"
"By *caring* for patients who suffer from asthma."
"Oh! I get it now. So you *do* treat asthma."
"No, I *don't.*"

Conversation with someone I know.

*When the name of a disease
becomes a stone wall.*

The name of a disease becomes a stone wall every day in
Star Wars Medicine (see the section on Star Wars Medicine).
At present, the name of the disease often serves as the magic
wand which swings to dissolve all rational thought about what
the true nature of a patient's suffering might be, how he could
go about relieving the various burdens on his biology, and what
options he might have in restoring his molecular and cellular
health.

GEORGIA'S STORY

Georgia, a Hispanic woman in her mid-forties, came to see
me one late evening in the middle of an asthma attack. She
had been treated for asthma in the intensive care unit of one
of our area hospitals and discharged three days earlier. The
asthma had returned. She told me this was her fourth hospital
admission for asthma during that year. During this time, and

several years before that, she had been treated with multiple drug therapies including steroids, evidently with poor results.

Georgia knew she had mold, pollen and food allergies. She also knew she was sensitive to many chemicals. Her allergies had not been investigated and treated. She had received neither any nutritional protocols nor any training for self-regulatory methods for control of her bronchial spasm.

She stayed in my office for about two hours that first evening. I was forced to give her adrenaline and benadryl injections. I used this time to explain to her how her asthma was being triggered by the various elements, and how we could systematically identify and eliminate these elements, and pursue the long-term goal of asthma control without any drugs.

I explained to her how the name of her disease (asthma) had become a *stone wall* for her.

We could accept this wall as the end of the world as the blind man did. We could try some other drug therapies. Or, we could choose a strategy for prevention and control of asthma with allergy desensitization, nutritional protocols for asthma, and *auto-regulation.* We could try to dissolve this *stone wall* as Dhobi dissolved his wall. I explained how we would not stop the use of drugs until such time that our allergy, nutritional and *auto-regulation* protocols make it unnecessary for us to use them. Georgia agreed. So we proceeded with the protocols for management of asthma.

In five months, I weaned her off steroids and all other

asthma drugs. Occasionally, she did experience some tightness in her chest and wheezing, but she had no difficulty controlling these symptoms with *auto-regulation*.

In self-regulation, a change in the perception of a disease leads to a change in the intensity of sufferings inflicted by it, and, with time, in healing.

Several weeks later, she returned with an asthma attack. Her pressure cooker had exploded setting fire to her kitchen. She simply could not control her asthma with *auto-regulation* this time. It has been more than eleven months since the kitchen fire. Georgia has neither used any drugs nor suffered from asthma attacks.

JANE'S STORY

Jane's case history was related to me by one of my internist-friends. Jane was hospitalized for asthma in one of the hospitals in New York City many years ago when my friend was in residency training.

Her asthma attack was brought under control with intravenous theophylline therapy. Soon after admission, Jane vomited some blood. The diagnostic work-up revealed what was thought to be a malignant lesion in her stomach. A biopsy was planned. Next day the chief of service conducted rounds accompanied by several residents and interns. He thought the stomach lesion was likely to be a cancer, and that she was much more likely to die of that cancer than her asthma. Unfortunately she learned about this. She developed another asthma attack which rapidly evolved into status asthmaticus (a condition of severe and unremitting spasm of bronchial tubes with progressive respiratory failure). She expired despite intensive and prolonged efforts to control status asthmaticus. At autopsy, no cancer was found in her stomach.

A CHILD WITH ASTHMA DIES

At times, I have had the saddening experience of performing an autopsy examination on patients who died with asthma. On one occasion, the patient was a young six year old boy. His face still showed the agony of struggle for breath, his skin blue with dark blood. His neck veins were distended. His lungs were ballooned out and filled with fluid. His bronchial tubes were clogged with mucus plugs.

Two days after I performed that autopsy, I went to Kansas

City to give a lecture on diagnosis and treatment of inhalant allergy and asthma in a post-graduate seminar organized by my close friend James Willoughby, M.D. of Liberty, Missouri. All during this seminar, I could not keep out of my mind the face of that little boy. The poor child was never investigated and treated for allergy.

"The mortality of asthma is low, averaging approximately 0.3 deaths per 100,000 persons. Typically, 2000 to 3000 people die of the disease per year, and the deaths tend to occur in the very young and in the elderly. The death rate from asthma may be increasing: data from 1983 and 1984 indicate an excess of 200 cases per year. The reasons for this purported increase are not clear. Some consider it to be artifactual, ------".

Pulmonary Diseases and Disorders
McGraw-Hill Book Company, 1988, page 1295

I have two comments.

First,

The mortality of asthma is *not* low for the parents of a single child who dies of asthma and who was never offered a chance to prevent asthma with treatment protocols of molecular medicine.

Second,

Before we consider the increase in the death rate from asthma as *artifactual,* we should first consider the essential issues of increasing sensitivity of asthma patients to environmental pollutants and foods and molds allergy.

WHAT ARE REALISTIC GOALS IN ASTHMA?

How often in clinical practice can one expect complete control over asthma with treatment protocols of molecular medicine (protocols for allergy, nutrition, fitness and *auto-regulation*) and without drugs?

The answer depends upon our knowledge of human biology and our philosophy of health and disease. A physician may consider asthma treatable only with drugs, prescribe theophylline, steroids or other drugs, and *prove* that asthma can be treated only with drugs. Or, a physician may consider asthma reversible, control asthma with molecular protocols, and *prove* that asthma is a reversible disorder.

In my experience, the answer is in the vast majority of

cases. Indeed, the few exceptions that I have seen are patients who suffered from severe concurrent immune disorders, patients with emphysema, and patients whose immune systems have been impaired with prolonged steroid therapy. Every attempt should be made to avoid steroids, except in the case of acute life-threatening emergencies. The short-term gains are not worth the huge price the patient pays over the long-haul.

In an *outcome* study we presented at the American Academy of Otolaryngic Allergy in January 1990, we reported our results with forty asthma patients who had been treated with standard drug therapies for a minimum period of one year before they consulted us, and for whom we had a minimum period of one year of follow-up. We were able to wean patients off their drugs completely in 72.5 %, and significantly reduce the drug use to occasional inhalations in another 15 % of patients. Only three patients (7.5 %) were still regularly using drugs at the end of the study period. See the section on *Lata and Limbic Breathing* for further details of this study.

I have seen laboratory evidence of allergy to mold in every single asthma patient I have treated. Food allergy and chemical sensitivity were almost always present. Pollen allergy was seen less often.

Asthma can be treated effectively without drugs with allergy and nutritional protocols. But, in my experience, the goal of *total control over asthma* will elude the patient until he learns to control the residual bronchial spasm with the methods of self-regulation.

There is still some uncertainty in the physician community about the role of allergy and nutritional protocols in the treatment of asthma. There are several reasons for this. First, physicians who specialize in lung disorders (pulmonolgists) generally are not trained to practice environmental medicine, nutritional medicine, and self-regulation. Second, many physicians continue to use various types of the RAST test which is not sufficiently sensitive to diagnosis all clinically significant mold allergy. This test is good for pollen allergy but misses up to one half of the mold sensitivity which can be diagnosed with the more advanced ELISA test. My research colleagues (Madhava Ramanarayanan, Ph.D. and others) and I documented this in a series of research reports. The professional reader may refer to the following publications for details.

Ali, M. et al. Am. J. Clinical Pathology 1984, 81: 591
Ali, M. et al. Am. J. Clinical Pathology 1983, 80: 290
Ali, M. et al. Annals of Allergy, 1980, 45: 63
Ali, M. et al. Clinical Allergy, 1980, 10: 203
Ali, M.   Clinical Ecology, 1986, 3: 68
Ali, M.   Otolaryngic Clinics of North America,
           1985, 18: 761
Ali, M.   Textbook of Otolaryngology and Head and Neck
           Surgery, Elsevier, New York, 1989. page 320

Recently some other researchers have drawn similar conclusions from their research studies.

"We conclude that asthma is almost always associated with some type of IgE-mediated (allergy) reaction."

New England Journal of Medicine
1989; 320:271

"-------, the bulk of the studies reviewed provide a strong suggestion that allergen immunotherapy in asthma is effective."

J. Allergy and Clinical Immunology
1989; 84: 137

Sometime ago I attended a medical conference. Three cases of asthma in young women were presented and discussed. All three patients were treated with the best tools of the Star Wars medicine in the intensive care unit. One of them developed a cardiac arrest, was coded, and fortunately survived.

The case discussions by two specialists included detailed descriptions of comprehensive batteries of blood gas studies and other lung function tests with computerized interpretations, multiple drug therapies, and sophisticated lung machine applications.

Not a single word was spoken about what might have

triggered asthma in these young women. There was no reference to allergy testing. There was no mention of any nutritional protocols. There were no deliberations of stress factors which might have precipitated the asthma attacks.

In another medical conference at our hospital, a guest speaker, a pulmonologist (lung specialist), lectured about asthma treatment for one hour. He discussed in detail the strengths and the weaknesses of a large number of drugs used for control of asthma. He described the adverse effects of various drugs and made recommendations about how to treat the side-effects of some drugs with yet other drugs.

Conspicuously missing from his presentation was any reference to allergy as the trigger for asthma. At the end of the lecture, one of our staff allergists asked him to comment on the role of allergy in asthma treatment and referred to the study published in the New England Journal of Medicine and cited previously. The speaker walked up to the seated allergist, gazed at him for a few moments, and then pronounced in a firm, authoritative tone,

" You must be an allergist. Right ! Right !! "

There was a polite laughter from the audience. The allergist smiled in embarrassment. All *good* speakers carry such quick verbal puns. You never know when you will need one.

Such verbal puns may be humorous and acceptable ways of

changing the subject, but it is not funny for a patient with asthma who cannot breathe, who is prescribed drugs, and who is denied the possibility of normal breathing without drugs.

MEDICINE IS A SELF-CORRECTING DISCIPLINE.

Science is self-correcting. Medicine is a branch of science. It follows that medicine must be self-correcting too, but medicine generally corrects itself slowly. Sometimes it moves painfully slowly for those who observe it. Often it moves maddeningly slowly for those in the captivity of chronic debilitating illnesses.

Rudolph Virchow, the German physician, philosopher, and statesman, published *cellular pathology* in 1858. He strived to liberate physicians of his time from the constraints of medieval and ancient ideas about gross pathology and disease. He did succeed, but it took many decades. Now we honor him as the father of modern pathology.

Much has changed since the time of Virchow. We developed technologies for sanitation and vaccination, and gained substantial survival advantages in our competitive struggle with the world of microbes. We became adept in the use of the surgical scalpel. We invented efficient ways of killing life around us with antibiotics, insecticides and pesticides. We brought upon ourselves chemical and electro-magnetic avalanches. We polluted out air and water. We contaminated our food with preservatives, pesticides, antibiotics and hormones. We speeded up life and accelerated aging. A state of *biologic burnout* became a *normal* state of the human condition.

Much has transpired since the time of Virchow. Our diseases have changed. Cellular pathology no longer gives us satisfactory clues to the initial molecular and electro-magnetic events which initiate disease and the cell membrane dynamics which perpetuate. Consider the causes of the major chronic, degenerative, metabolic, autoimmune, and allergic disorders. We recognize we do not know the true causes of any of these disorders. Still, we cling to the Virchonian ideas of cellular pathology. Like other major intellectual adaptations, the change from cellular and molecular thinking will take time.

The nimble-footed in medicine

Medicine does move quickly in some areas. We physicians seem to be quite nimble-footed when it comes to new drugs or new surgical procedures. We respond well to the power and persuasiveness of our drug industry. The acceptance of new drugs and new surgical procedures by the Star Wars medical community appears to occur at the speed of lightning. The glamor of the Star Wars technology is too much to resist for any *progressive* physician.

We, physicians as well as patients, seem to have literally taken to heart the advice of an old physician who observed,

"Use a new drug early while it works."

This old physician had a rare insight into how drugs really work. We seem not to recognize it.

"The fact is, we're all depressed. The whole world is depressed. I don't know a human being who isn't," says one doctor. Which raises the question, should everyone take Prozac?"

New York magazine   Dec. 18, 1989 page 50

Pull of the Possibilities

I started my work in pathology in 1968. In 1974, I was asked to serve as the Director of the Department of Pathology, Immunology and Laboratories at Holy Name Hospital, Teaneck, New Jersey. From 1971 to 1984, I co-authored 11 pathology books with my associate pathologists, Evalynne Braun, M.D. and Alfred Fayemi, M.D. (Dr. Fayemi is now Chief of Pathology at St. Mary's Hospital, Hoboken, N.J.) These books were written to help pathologists in residency training to prepare for their Specialty Board Examination. During this time, I also co-authored with my colleagues over 75 research papers. These early *formative* years were busy years. It was a period of an intensive study of the various disciplines of pathology which included general pathology, immunology, surgical pathology, autopsy pathology, hematology, clinical chemistry, immunochemistry, and microbiology. Of course, writing pathology books was an academic interest for my associate pathologists and I. Our day's work was still the work of a hospital pathologist: microscopic diagnosis of biopsies and surgical specimens, autopsy examinations, and analysis in the clinical laboratory.

How do diseases begin?

What is the true nature of diseases? How is a state of

health replaced with a state of disease ? What are the initial molecular and electro-magnetic events which change a healthy cell to a diseased cell ? How do molecules age ? How do molecules get sick ? These were the questions which preoccupied my mind during this period.

With passing years, I became increasingly doubtful of the validity of many of our prevailing ideas about naming and classifying diseases. I developed a growing awareness of the impact of poor nutrition, food and mold allergy, environmental sensitivity, stress, and problems of physical fitness on human health. These were the molecular burdens on biology. Diseases, it appeared to me, were the consequence of these burdens, often unrecognized or neglected. Even the growing menace of recurrent viral infections and parasitic infestations was clearly the result of an impaired immune system.

What if one could keep one's focus on the molecular and electro-magnetic events which initiate cell injury ? What if one could stay with the cell membrane dynamics which perpetuate cell injury ? What if one could move away from disease names when these names do not give us any insight into the nature of what ails a patient ? What if one could systematically identify and address all the burdens on a patient's biology? What if one could base all treatment strategies on these considerations ? What if one could stay with molecules which are well-known to human biology (nutrients and plant derivatives) ? What if one could stay away from what is unknown to our biology (synthetic drugs)?

Such thinking is generally regarded as simple-mindedness. Impractical and removed from real life! That is how such thoughts are dismissed. I recognized this. Yet I could not keep such thoughts out of my mind.

The pull of such possibilities was simply too great for me.

A time to listen to some patients.
A time to close my books.

This was my considered decision when I started my clinical work with a handful of patients with severe immune disorders. This seems bizarre now, but it seemed very logical then.

After I stopped my work on pathology books, a lot of time became available to me. I was ready to test my ideas about human biology and disease which had been incubating in my mind during the years I was doing research and writing pathology and immunology books. My interest and research in immunology, in particular, seemed to pull me ever more strongly to a basic but scientifically sound treatment approach based on concepts of molecular medicine (nutritional medicine, environmental medicine, and medicines of fitness, and self-regulation).

My early patients were a handful of very sick patients disillusioned with multiple failures of antibiotics, cortisone treatment, and other prevailing drug therapies. They were quite willing to test this possibility with me. The idea of closing my books and listening to them, after all, did not seem so *far-out*.

Biologic Burnout

So this is how I set out to face what I had regarded as a state of " Biologic Burnout" in these patients. Availability of ample time and freedom from immediate need for research funding seem to set the stage. What was required was full knowledge for the patient and persistence on my part. I was prepared, I thought.

I have described the evolution of my thoughts about the principles and practice of self-regulation and molecular medicine in the section on *Ten Lessons Learned From Patients*. In the companion volumes *The Dog and the Dis-ease Syndrome* and *The Pheasant and Suffering in Illness*, I relate some of my early personal observations with methods of self-regulation and other treatment protocols of molecular medicine.

CHANTING IN A BOARD ROOM

Self-regulation and healing has always held a great interest for man. Throughout history, and in particular in the Sumerian,

Egyptian, Indian, Tibetan, Greco-Roman, and more recently in medieval cultures, men of medicine and men of letters showed an abiding interest in methods of self-regulation. The methods for self-healing and the meditative techniques of the Egyptian priests, Hindu yogis, Tibetan lamas, Greco-Roman physicians, and Muslim dervishes, have all been well-documented.

How does a young American woman, incarcerated in her house with disabling chronic fatigue, relate to meditative techniques of Tibetan lamas in Himalayan mountains ? How does an American child with Tourette's syndrome or hyperactivity practice the methods of a Muslim dervish to control a metabolic roller-coaster caused by food allergy, bad nutrition, and stress ? How does an American executive with high blood pressure, daily headaches, and a stomach ulcer engage in a yogi's chants in a board-room ?

In Auto-regulation, healing comes through regulation of biology. It comes with changes in molecules, cells, and tissues caused with deliberate efforts, with knowledge and insight.

I wanted to explore the methods which would help my patients achieve this goal. I wanted methods which would be practical and relevant for the modern man.

I had good reasons to listen to my patients, and keep my

books closed.

TECHNOLOGIES FOR SELF-REGULATION CHANGE; PRINCIPLES OF SELF-REGULATION DO NOT.

The science and technology of modern medicine have made it possible for any person to clearly see and know his disease at microscopic, electro-physiologic, and molecular levels. This is not science fiction. It is a simple concept which we use in our *auto-regulation* protocols every day.

A person can know his disease at a microscopic level with accurate microscopic imaging. For various diseases, I teach patients disease-specific imaging using microscopic pictures of the body organ in disease. Patient see the damaged tissues in the disease state in true-to-life images.

A person can know his disease at an electro-physiologic level with his own "Biologic Profile", a dynamic and moving composite picture of graphs showing the state of his internal body organs on a computer screen. In our auto-regulation laboratory, I show patients how they can alter their own biologic profiles with simple exercises.

A person can know his disease at a molecular level with a study of his own living cells as they react to different molecules. I show this to our patients with high resolution video technology.

Injured molecules, cells and tissues, all heal with energy. Auto-regulation is about this energy.

Different technologies offer different advantages. What needs to be held constant is a clear view of our goals: an awareness of the energy in our tissues; a desire to attend to our tissues; and *listening for healing* rather than *talking for control.*

Beyond positive thinking: Two states of the human condition.

Early in my work with *auto-regulation*, I learned from my patients a useful (and now clinically validated) conceptual model for self-healing. In this model, we see human biology in two conditions. First is the   condition of biology which is created and sustained by a part of our brain (the neo-cortex) which calculates, computes, competes, cautions, and clutters our minds. I call this the " *cortical mode* ". The second condition of biology is created and sustained by a part of the brain (the limbic system) which cares, comforts and consoles. I call this the " *limbic mode* ".

I learned by personal experience and by working with my patients that it is extremely difficult, if at all possible, to be aware of, to become sensitive to, and to regulate our biology when we are in the *cortical mode.* To do so, one needs to learn how to escape into the *limbic mode.*

Positive thinking, as desirable as it may seem, is still thinking. My work with very ill patients has convinced me that positive thinking alone is not sufficient to change a biology in turbulence into a biology in a calm, steady and regenerative state. Positive thinking, under these circumstances, is generally nothing but a euphemism, often a cruel play on words for the patient in unremitting suffering.

The Cortical Mode

The *cortical mode*   counts, computes, and competes. It censors and cautions. It controls and constricts. It assesses and analyzes. It wavers and warns. It gives us chronic thinking. And with its unrelenting chatter, it causes stress,impaired immunity and leads to *The Dis-ease Syndrome. The Dis-ease Syndrome,* if not reversed, damages tissues and causes disease. I discuss these issues in the companion volume *The Dog and the Disease Syndrome*.

The Limbic Mode

By contrast, the *limbic mode* cares and comforts. It soothes and pampers. It gives and accepts affection and love. It creates images of health. It heals.

In this mode, our biology is in a steady state, assuring the continuity in basic life functions. It keeps in order the rhythm of the heart, arterial pulses, muscle tone, breathing cycles, and other essential life functions.

In this healing model, these two states of the human condition are held in balance and harmony to preserve health. But the problems of modern life (stress, poor nutrition, and sensitivity to environmental pollution) disrupt this balance and harmony. The *cortical brain* often suppresses the *limbic brain*.In patients with severe dysfunctions, the suppression of the *limbic brain* may be so complete as to paralyze it.

I discuss this concept of the two states of human biology in detail in the section on *Beyond Positive Thinking: Two States of the Human Condition* in the companion volume *The Pheasant and Suffering in Illness*.

Legacy of Dhobidharma

The legacy of Dhobidharma to us is this:

* We can look at the name of a chronic disease
  as the blind man looked at his stone wall, limit
  ourselves by it, and set the stage for a long-term
  chemical dependence on drugs.

Or,

* We can look at the name of a chronic disease as
  Dhobi looked at his stone wall, learn to dissolve
  it, and set the stage for freedom from the disease
  and dependence on drugs.

****

*Men occasionally stumble over
the truth, but most of them
pick themselves and hurry off
as if nothing happened.*

Winston Churchill

Section 2

Ten Lessons
Learned From Patients

The task of science is to stake out the limits of the knowable, and to center consciousness within them.

Rudolph Virchow
Father of pathology

My approach to *auto-regulation* as a model for self-healing, and the methods of *auto-regulation* evolved over a period of several years. During this time, I spent long hours listening to my patients and observing their biology. The concepts and methods of *auto-regulation* are based much more on what their biology taught me, and much less on what I thought of their diseases. The principles underlying this model, however, are time-honored and represent our Eastern and Western cultural heritage.

*Serendipity rather than any clever
design led me to Auto-regulation.*

I wanted to be a surgeon long before I entered medical school. If this was ever a considered decision, I do not remember. A career in medicine carried the promise of caring for those in pain and illness. Physicians were held in high esteem in Pakistan in those days. None of them carried an aura around them the way surgeons did. I suppose that seemed enough to a young boy in high school.

After my medical education, I trained as a house-surgeon at Mayo Hospital, Lahore. Surgery was my consuming passion. I recall discussing the choice of a surgical career with one of my professors. When asked why he became a surgeon, his reply was quick,

"Because I love the smell of human blood."

I do not know if he was trying to amuse me. But I do remember that his response seemed genuine to me. It seemed to be an answer that I would have wanted to give if I had been asked the question. I often remember this conversation for it clearly brings back to me those heady early surgery days when I was a servant, and the surgical scalpel my master.

A world of human organs

After my work at Mayo Hospital, I continued my surgical training, first in Swansea, Wales, and then in London. I passed the examination and received the diploma of a Fellow of the Royal College of Surgeons of England. In 1966, I came to this country for what I thought was going to be a year of surgical residency, my introduction to the American way of "doing it".

My year of surgical residency at the Jersey City Medical Center was unrewarding. In England, I had the opportunity to work at a senior level, make some decisions and participate in others, and often operate on my own. In Jersey city, I had no say in the making of surgical decisions. Essentially I served as a mechanical device employed by junior residents. In surgical parlance, it is called "holding retractors", which means keeping tissues out of the way of the operating surgeon. I knew this was the price every foreign surgeon had to pay (and rightfully so) for coming to the US. Still it did not spare me the boredom of entry level surgical "scut work". The fact that I had accepted this position knowing all this did not help me either. My mind wandered a lot in that year.

Surgical pathology in Pakistan in those years was a nonexistent specialty. The path reports came to us weeks after the surgery. The patients, by then, were usually lost to the followup. Even when we did see the patients on re-visits, the path report was not a high priority. Our professors did not seem to have much confidence in the pathologist's interpretations. I thought of spending a year in a pathology residency before returning to Pakistan for a career in general surgery. May be that would help, I reasoned.

A world of Cells

The microscope opened up for me the "divine Disneyland" of the human tissues. The Disneyland of biology is limitless.For a young curious mind, a microscope has no match. Surgical training had given me a feel for the living organs; the microscope gave me windows to the world of tissues and cells. Surgical pathology quickly replaced surgery as my current passion. There were still more turns to come in my work, but my involvement with the microscope to this day has been a lasting affair.

Like most young pathologists, my early research projects and papers were in the field of cancer. The search for the cause of cancer, and the potential for cure, fascinates people in and out of medicine alike. Cancer is not one disease. Some cancers are rabid; they have voracious appetite for tissue destruction and sharp instincts for distant strikes. Other cancers are subdued in their growth. So we are not going to eventually settle with one cause and one cure. This is the single most important insight I obtained from my personal involvement in this area.

Cancer is the consequence of environmental impact on the genetic make-up of an individual. Since a change in the genetic make-up of a person is not possible at this time, the only valid strategy for protection from this dread disease is to look at the environmental factors and immune defenses (nutrition, stress, sensitivity to chemical pollutants, viral infections, and what I call in this book the *cortical Living)*.

A world of molecules

Growing, aging, hurting and healing, all are expressions of molecular dynamics.

Young women and men of medicine go to pathology for the microscope; the requirements of a modern laboratory push them to diagnostic analyses. The field of testing and analysis is called clinical pathology. My appointment as the director of laboratories at Holy Name Hospital, Teaneck in 1974 required that I become a clinical pathologist. This had not been my considered choice, but it appeared to be necessary at that time.

The world of molecules is different from the world of organs and the world of cells. I fell in love with this world. Blood is a vast cosmos of molecules. There are so many things one can measure in blood. The laboratory became one huge toy store for the boy in me. My research interests expanded to include some projects about early diagnosis of myocardial infarction (heart attack), liver disease, and lung disorders.

A world of crisis

During my four years of residency in pathology, first at Holy Name Hospital and later at Columbia Presbyterian

Hospital in New York, I moonlighted as an emergency room physician. Most foreign doctors had to do so to support their families. The emergency work at St. James Hospital in Newark and then at Irvington General Hospital in Irvington was often gruelling (coming as it did after a day's work in the pathology department). This work was also very rewarding. Heart attacks and life-threatening trauma have a way of stripping people of all pretensions. These are times for being truthful, for the patient, for the family, and for those who minister to them.

Emergency medicine is also a time to watch our therapies misfire. There were days when I watched in frustration my treatment fail my patients in the emergency room during the night hours, and then studied the causes of such therapeutic failures in the autopsy room during the day hours.

A world of the teachers and pupils

My appointment on the faculty of Columbia University assured me continued access to many of the most gifted teachers and researchers in the field of pathology. It also rendered me vulnerable to the raw prying minds of doctors in the making. Medical students have a way of asking the most disconcerting questions. Unrestrained by the contingencies of clinical medicine, these students wanted to know more about where the disease begins, rather than how to treat advanced disease.

The legacy of my students is this: while our knowledge of the cellular basis of disease has grown enormously in recent decades, our understanding of the molecular and electro-magnetic events which initiate cellular injury is still very limited. Indeed, medical texts are replete with description of diseases and syndrome for which the initial cause is unknown. These include premature aging, almost all immune disorders (autoimmune and immune deficiencies), degenerative diseases, and cancer.

A world of a "new biology"

In the late sixties, Sr. Patricia Lynch, the president of our hospital foresaw the need for a new service at the hospital. She invited my close friend Robert Rigolosi,M.D. to organize a regional dialysis center at the hospital. This center soon grew into the largest dialysis facility in the State. Dr. Rigolosi is a man deeply committed to his patients and his work. He has been relentless in his search for answers, even to that last court of appeal: the autopsy examination. The autopsy rate for our dialysis patients during the first ten years ranged from 80-90% We realized that we had access to more pathologic material than most other pathology groups. This led to the publication of our book " Pathology of Maintenance Dialysis" in 1982. I co-authored this book with my associate pathologist, Alfred O. Fayemi,M.D.

Our research in the pathology of chronic dialysis, and extensive literature review undertaken in the preparation of our book, was a prolonged and a very unusual educational experience. We were fortunate to develop clinically useful new information in many areas. But it was much more than that.

Month by month, I came to recognize the changing character of what we thought was "proven knowledge". The change from the established "proven knowledge" to the new knowledge is often quite unsettling, even for the "open-minded" in medicine.

Chronic dialysis, by prolonging life with the "kidney machine", has created a "new biology" for the man living without kidneys.

Before we can learn this "new biology", we need to unlearn the "old biology". This is not an easy task. I will cite one small example.

One of our research project concerned iron storage and transport in chronic hemodialysis patients. We observed heavy iron deposits in the liver and absence of iron in the bone marrow of many patients. Normally, iron is present in appreciable quantities only in the bone marrow where it is used to make hemoglobin in red blood cells. This was an obvious paradox: iron was absent from the bone marrow where it was needed, and it was present in excess in the liver where it was causing liver injury.

We published our initial observations in the Journal of American Medical Association (Ali, M. et al, 244:343-

345,1980).

As simple as this observation appeared to be, it challenged the validity of many aspects of the then "proven knowledge" about iron metabolism. We made some further observation about ferritin (one of the major proteins which carries iron) in blood in a more extensive follow-up study. This second study validated our conclusions drawn from the first study and raised some new questions about the "proven" knowledge in this area. The paper written to publish the results of this study was rejected by eleven medical journals. The response letter from a major journal included the following comment, "The implications of this paper will radically change our ideas about iron storage and transport." Fully recognizing that the microscopic and chemical observations being reported in our paper were important, the journal rejected the paper. Our paper was finally published in the British journal The Lancet (Ali, M. et al i:652-655, 1982). Our observations have been confirmed by several other investigators since.

When kidneys fail, the dialysis patients face sudden and drastic changes in their biology. These changes are easy to see and quantify. But how does biology change when the changes in our external environments and internal homeostasis are insidious in onset and slow to evolve? Our research studies in the pathology of dialysis brought me some important insights in biology.

First,

Biology is forever changing; we change one thing in

one way, we change everything in some way.

Second,

Medicine is forever self-correcting. Self-corrections in medicine, however, are in general very slow to take form.

Third,

The initial response of women and men in medicine to new observations invalidating "proven" knowledge is more often than not a simple denial.

Fourth,

True science is search for truth. Since biology is a changing science, truth in biology must be accepted as intrinsically changing.

A world of the immune system

Immunity is an organism's ability to preserve its health. Immunology is the medical specialty which deals with disorders of immunity. Pathology is the study of disease. Immunology and pathology, thus, are the flip sides of the same coin. All practicing pathologists eventually become closet immunologists. Pathology, in essence, is the study of the immune system. I did not stay a closet immunologist for too long. My fascination with the immune system was irrepressible.

Windows on the world

Man has two windows on the world around him:

1. *The human brain*
2. *The human immune system*

We take evident pride in our minds. At a superficial level, our brain does seem to influence and determine all aspects of our existence. Man can think and scribe. So he considers himself to be a rational and a social being. We seem to believe that our brains differentiate us from the rest of the animal kingdom. We attribute to our brains all our successes. From a biologic perspective, this view is simplistic and very restricted.

The second window of the immune system is infinitely more important to the survival of man as a species. What separates us from other forms of life around us, and indeed from each other, is the uniqueness of the molecules and cells of the immune system. These molecules and cells *"think"*, and distinguish between the *"self"* and *"non-self"*. The immune system forever seeks to preserve the Self within the organism and obliterate the Non-self. Man's feats of intellect can take form only because his immune system allows him to preserve his structural integrity, and pursue intellectual goals. Health is a preserve, first of the immune system, and only then of the brain.

The immune system is creativity of Nature at its best. There are the B-lymphocyte cells, the immune cells which produce antibodies. There are the T-lymphocytes which regulate the structure, growth, and function of B-cells. There are T cells which are helpful (the helper T-cells). Then there are T cells which hold back the B-cells (the suppressor T-cells). There are the Null cells which defy any visible purpose. There are Natural Killer cells which kill by innate instincts and need no programming. There are molecules which carry messages to other cells (Lymphokines), and other molecules which provide docking sites on the surface membranes of the immune cells(membrane receptors). When called upon, the immune cells even produce hormones. These molecules and cells do not live in isolation; indeed, these are pieces of Nature's molecular balancing acts, an ever-changing kaleidoscope of molecular alignments and re-alignments. Immunology, then, is the first discipline among medical disciplines.

A world of psycho-neuro-immunology

There is a new area of medical inquiry. It concerns the interface of the known and measurable physical-chemical aspects of our biology (the body) and the as yet unknown and immeasurable physical-chemical aspects of our biology (the mind). In the scientific terminology, it is called *psycho-neuro-*

immunology. There has been an explosion of new knowledge in this burgeoning new medical field. Children have been taught to raise the levels of protective antibodies in their blood with imaging methods. The number of immune cells in blood has been increases by harnessing the healing power of the mind. Positive skin tests produced by injection of allergens in the skin have been turned negative with meditation techniques. I cite many more specific examples of these phenomena in other chapters of this book.

A world of nutrition and chemical sensitivity

I started my work in allergy, sensitivity to environmental agents, and nutrition after several years of research and practice in the fields of pathology, immunology, and allergy. The publication of my research papers in allergy and immunology brought me many invitations to present my research data at national medical conferences. On these occasions, I had the good fortune to meet many physicians with extraordinary insights into the matters of health and disease. During meal times and cocktail hours, they related to me case histories of patients who were clearly sensitive to foods, molds and environmental pollutants. Yet these patients did not fit any descriptions in the medical texts. When faced with information like that, our tendency generally is to dismiss the whole circumstance as apocryphal. I chose to doubt the veracity of neither these physicians nor their patients.

These physicians often queried me about the immunologic

basis of such illnesses. These were evidently difficult questions. There were no ready answers. But the questions would stay with me.

I was being prepared, it seems. Prepared for what? For self-regulation!! This thought never crossed my mind.

The very term self-healing, after all, was heretical in the professional circles I was in. The term self-regulation, quite evidently, is a polite euphemism for self-healing. The best way to preserve my scientific standing, I had been advised, was to keep my distance from "unproven" methods. That always raised an interesting question for me.

If everybody was to keep away from these "unproven" methods, how would these methods ever get proven?

A world of self-healing

My early patients in my work with immune disorders consulted me for two main reasons. First, they suffered from complex, chronic and indolent diseases. The prevailing standard methods of treatment for their immune dysfunctions had not been successful after multiple trials. Second, they were either family members or close friends of my professional associates, and were familiar with my fairly extensive research and teaching experiences in these areas.

As I searched for methods to treat these patients, I knew I was groping in the dark. I also knew that there was a good chance I would not succeed. But this did not create any ethical problems for me. I found it simple and easy to explain the true state of affairs to these patients. I also decided not to bill these patients for my services until I was in a position to predict in some way the outcome of my efforts.

Some of these patients had been on the verge of utter helplessness. They had previously undergone extensive diagnostic testing and received multiple drug therapies without clinical benefit. They were very grateful that I was willing to work with them. They fully understood that my efforts might not prove more rewarding than those made earlier by others.

These few early patients taught me ten essential lessons. The story of *auto-regulation* is the story of these lessons.

FIRST LESSON:
Words are codes for images.

"Healing " is a word which carries, for a physician, certain images of diagnosis and drugs. It gives him some ideas about the probability of success.

"Self-healing" is a word which carries, for a patient, no images of his body organ in disease. It gives him neither any images for reversing the disease process nor any clear idea of the probability of success.

But what if this were changed? What if the word "self-healing" carried for the patient accurate and precise images of his body organ in disease? What if this word brought to him clear images for reversing the disease process without drugs? Could self-healing, then, take place? My patients speaking in this book give eloquent answers to this question.

I am by calling a dealer in words and words are, of course, the most powerful drugs used by mankind.

Kipling,
in a speech to the Royal College of Surgeons

One only sees what one looks for, one only looks for what one knows.

Goethe

LIZ, MY TEACHER

I have been a student of medicine for over 32 years. The single most important lesson I learned in these years was taught to me by Liz.

Liz is a high school drop out who works as a hair dresser in our town. Liz had suffered from migraine for several years.She came to see me in the throes of a severe attack which had lasted for three days. She had vomited several times that day, was obviously dehydrated, and was running a fever of 101.5 degrees. After clinical evaluation, I felt compelled to give her a strong pain-killer by injection to control her migraine on this first visit.

During her second visit next day, her head still hurt, though not so intensely as it did the night before. I explained to her the probable causes of her migraine, and the likely role of spasms of her blood vessels in her head. We went to our *auto-reg* laboratory. I attached to her arms sensors for electronic equipment for various electro-physiological parameters. I recorded some baseline readings and then took Liz through some of our basic training in *auto-reg* methods. It is not unusual for me to observe some patients make significant progress during the very first training session in our *auto-reg* lab. The electro-physiologic responses seen are dramatic, and the documentation on the computer screen most revealing to the patient. On some occasions, such responses seem miraculous. Liz turned out to be one such example.

The graphs of her heart and arteries on the computer screen displayed sharp and dramatic changes. I froze the computer screen and asked her how she felt and if her headache was in any way different. She seemed puzzled for a few moments and then spoke with obvious joy,

" It is gone,"

I explained to her the significance of what had happened. I talked about what the graphs indicated and interpreted the changes she caused in them by her *auto-regulation* exercises. She listened to me intently, thought for a few moments, and then said,

"Are you saying I changed those graphs with my mind?"
"Yes!," I replied.
"You mean you did not change the sensitivity on the
computer!" she asked.
"No," I responded.

Liz leaned back on her chair, and stared at me blankly. At length she spoke,

"You mean it was in me all this time to open my arteries
and control my migraine. You mean I just did not know
it. I suffered all these years and took all those drugs

for no reason."

"I never looked at it in that light, Liz. But it does seem so," I replied.

I knew what Liz meant. I myself suffered from severe migraine headaches for 35 years. Since my migraine attacks never responded to any pain pills, I was forced to take injections of demerol. During my early clinical work with self-regulation, I had learned to dissolve my headaches with *auto-regulation*. I knew Liz like me was going to resolve this problem once and for all. It is over two years since I first saw Liz. She regularly controls her headaches with *auto-regulation* and without drugs. The migraine is gone.

The lesson taught to me by Liz was simple:

We can arrest the course of a disease, and with time, reverse it if only we can know it at a biologic-intuitive level.

This is the core idea of *auto-regulation*. First, we know what is hidden under our skin. Second, we become sensitive to it. Third, we learn to regulate it. And finally, we use these insights and skills to reverse disease and heal ourselves.

SECOND LESSON
Our biology never lies to us,
nor does it ever accept lies from us.

I have never seen a patient who could trick his own heart, deceive his own brain, fool his own arteries, fake his own glands, malign his own muscles, or sham his own skin.

My body respond to me;
my genes wrote, but I can change in many
ways, the blue-print of my biology.

If we can see clearly the form and function of a body organ in health, and if we can see how it becomes different when it is in distress, we can affect a change in it, first in its function, then in its form.

A patient with heart palpitations slows down his heart rate and one with irregular rhythm corrects his rhythm. A patient switches off a sensitivity reaction provoked by an exposure to a chemical. A hyperactive child turns off a reaction caused by food allergy. A patient with migraine headache relieves his headache attack. A patient with asthma attack controls his wheezing attack. A patient with hypertension normalizes his blood pressure. These are some of the results our patients have achieved with *auto-regulation*.

Each one of these patients bears testimony to the link between our insights in biology and regulation of the function, and with time, the structure of our body organs.

The reach of self-healing with *auto-regulation* goes far beyond some selected case histories. See the section on *The Cortical Monkey and Healing* and the companion volume *The Pheasant and Suffering in Illness*.

THIRD LESSON
People in self-healing intuitively respond to their biologic profiles.

The issue today is not that people do not want self-healing; the issue is that they do not know *how* to heal themselves without drugs and without a surgeon's scalpel.

In *auto-regulation*, we approach this problem of *how to* by teaching patients simple methods for observing and exploring their biology. We use the term "Biologic Profile" for a composite pictures which graphically demonstrate to the patient the structure and function of his various body tissues.

These biologic profiles are true-to-life, precise and accurate images of electro-magnetic, molecular, and microscopic events which occur in a patient's biology in health and disease. Our technology allows us to look at living cells, tissues, and organs. In my own clinical work I focus on those methods where a person can see what is abnormal, respond to it, and then see for himself the effects of his efforts. Other technologies such as pictures of ovaries taken with a laparoscope (an instrument used to examine the inside of the belly) or snap-shots of stomach ulcer taken with a gastroscope are also very useful even though these are not suitable for seeing immediate responses to methods of self-regulation.

A biologic profile of a patient may consist of moving integrated graphs showing the activity of various body organs. We describe for our patients the significance of each of the components in these profiles. We ask our patients to observe their own profiles. We explain to them the meanings of each of the elements of these graphs. Next, we teach them simple methods for affecting a change in the functions of these organs. This is followed by instruction in the specific methods for treating specific diseases. In essence, this is what we mean by observation and exploration of biology.

The biologic profile for a patient may be limited and confined to two or three body organs, or it may be comprehensive and integrate the details of several organs simultaneously on a single computer screen. Specifically, biologic profiles can be designed to include the heart rate and rhythm, patterns of circulation, activity in different parts of the brain, electrical charges in the muscles, and levels of energy (galvanic or conductance) in skin responses. An examples of a biologic profile follows:

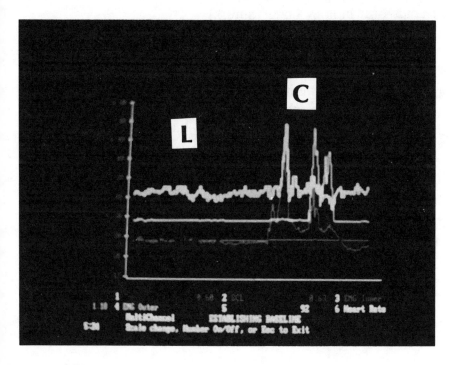

The biologic profile shown above graphically demonstrates how a person can change his biology from a turbulent Cortical mode to an even *limbic mode* with *auto-reg*. The graph lines on the computer screen reflect the activities of the heart, arterial pulses, skin conductance energy, and electrical activity in muscles. The right side of the computer screen, indicated by letter C, shows a biology in the *cortical mode*. The various organ function graphs display tall peaks and deep lows (loud signals of a biology under duress).

The left side of the computer screen, indicated by letter L, shows a biology in the *limbic mode*. The electro-physiologic indicators of the activities of the various body organs show smooth even lines indicating a calm steady state of biology. What separated these two states of biology was the practice of *auto-regulation* methods for about seven minutes.

The message given by this biologic profile to its owner, the patient wired to the computer screen with electronic sensors, is simple, loud, and clear. The way he attends to his own *cortical* (intellectual) thoughts or listens to (and responds) to his tissues determines the state of his biology.

He has a choice:

He can choose the cortical mode, keep his biology in turbulence, and perpetuate his disease, or

*He can choose the limbic mode, keep
his biology at an even pace, and self-heal.*

*"Of all the strange features of the
universe, none are stranger than these:
time is transcended, laws are mutable,
and observer participancy matters."*

John Wheeler, Professor of physics
Princeton University

On other occasions, I use biologic profiles which are composed of dynamic moving microscopic pictures of blood cells or other tissues, projected on a video screen and enlarged 10-15 thousand times. Such true-to-life pictures literally allow the person to get into her blood stream or tissues to observe the scene in living details, an *in the body experience*. An example of such a profile follows:

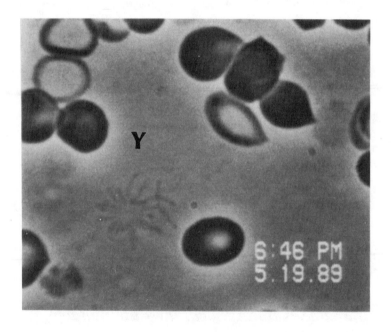

The biologic profile shown above belongs to a woman who suffered from asthma for many years inspite of multiple drug therapy. She was having 8-10 asthma attacks daily and required frequent use of medication. I had treated her successfully with allergy desensitization, nutritional protocols, and Auto-reg methods so that she became free of both asthma and drugs. Now she returned with repeated asthma attacks. She had missed several injections and had not been taking nutritional protocols which I had prescribed. Her blood profile (given above) shows some deformed red blood cells, some clumped red cells, and a colony of yeast cells (indicated by letter Y). The yeast colony actually moved like an octopus while she and I watched it on the video screen.

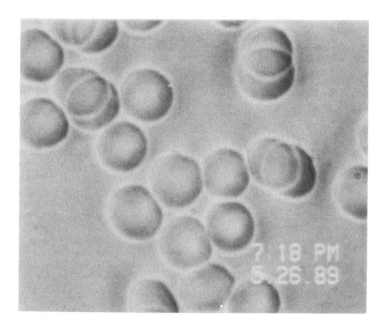

The blood profile shown above belongs to the same woman

and was taken one week later. This profile shows healthy red blood cells with regular smooth cell membranes. Healthy cells carry a negative surface charge (symbolically shown by the glow of refracted light in the picture). The cells show no clumping. There are no yeast cells.

She was treated with protocols for intravenous and oral nutritional supplements, allergy desensitization injections, nystatin to control yeast growth, and Auto-reg methods. I did not prescribe any drugs to control her bronchospasm (wheezing). At the time of repeat profiling, she had been completely free of asthma attacks, and had stopped using all drugs for asthma.

What role did these profiles play in her recovery? Without these profiles, my explanations about her ailment would have been theoretical and abstract. Actual blood profiles, done at the time of uncontrollable asthma and again after asthma had been controlled, gave her irrefutable evidence for a biologic change which had been brought about by our treatment approach. This *in the body experience* was an essential part of her self-healing, even though we may not fully understand the dynamics involved in this at present.

In *auto-regulation*, we use a person's own biologic profile as the centerpiece of our program for teaching him control and regulation of his body organ functions. We begin with simple tasks such as slowing the heart rate, increasing blood circulation to hands, and changing the patterns of brain waves. Next, we move on to training in *disease-specific auto-reg*. Here again, these biologic profiles usually provide the best possible forms of true-to-life imaging.

A print-out of a biologic profile, taped to a wall in work area or a kitchen wall is very useful. It assists the patient in knowing his disease at a biologic-intuitive level.

The essential value of this approach to self-healing is this: a person's own biologic profile, and the changes he can make in this profile by his own willful efforts, allow him to break through the barriers of disbelief about self-healing. I have observed this phenomenon most dramatically in children. Children are natural *auto-reggers*.

FOURTH LESSON
Self-regulation cannot be a purely intellectually pursuit; healing cannot be forced upon our tissues when we are in the "Cortical Mode". It happens when we listen to them in the "Limbic Mode".

The first core idea of *auto-regulation* requires that the

patient fully understand the nature of his disease; the second, that he begin to explore his biology, learn to regulate his body organs, and finally reverse his disease process and self-heal. It requires a shift from the usual mind-set of wanting control over our circumstances (*the cortical mode*) to one of insight and harmony with our biology (the Limbic mode). The *cortical* mode is the thinking mode. The *limbic mode* is the feeling (and healing) mode. The difference between these two modes is very real and critical to success in self-healing. See the section on *Beyond Positive Thinking: A Concept of Two States of the Human Condition* in the companion volume *The Pheasant and Suffering in Illness.*

In our *Auto-regulation* laboratory, I have observed, predictably and reproducibly, how the manner by which a person attends to his own thoughts and feelings determines the state of his biology. He stresses his biology when he enters the *cortical mode*. He calms and rests his biology when he settles into the *limbic mode*. We have a choice:

We can perpetuate a chronic illness by speaking about it, forever analyzing it, and suppressing its symptoms with drugs.

or

We can heal an illness by listening to our biology, responding to it, and regulating it.

The Western culture, in some ways, can be seen as a culture of confession. We often believe that to speak is to heal. To name a disease is to understand it. To classify a disease is to conquer it. To use drugs for a disease is to cure it. This model served us well when we fought against polio, small pox and other infectious diseases. But is it applicable to the vast majority of diseases we fight today? Is the "cure with a drug" model relevant to illnesses caused by problems of nutrition, stress, environmental pollutants, and fitness?

Self-regulation offers a person an alternative. It offers a choice between speaking and drugging for control of disease and listening and responding for insight and healing.

FIFTH LESSON:
Self-healing cannot be dispensed by a prescription pad. The professional must first learn it himself, with insight and patience. Then he can teach it to his patients, with care and compassion.

Self-healing cannot be a clinical-analytical prescription. It is one thing to rationally and intellectually understand how a disease process causes pain and suffering. It is an altogether different matter to learn how to reverse that disease process with self-healing. If the two were the same, physicians themselves would heal their own stomach ulcers and normalize their high blood pressure without drugs. They would not use drugs for their children and spouses as the treatment of choice for chronic problems.

Personal observations with the methods of self-healing are essential for the professional teaching it to his patients.

In *auto-regulation*, the focus is on measurable changes in biologic aspects brought about with deliberate effort. The goal is a learned ability for regulating body functions. Healing occurs as a consequence. The physician is a tutor, and the patient, a student. We cannot teach anything well to others if we do not know it well ourselves.

A teacher must first enhance his own awareness of his biology, by listening to it, by exploring it, by learning to regulate it. For instance, a physician cannot hope to teach a patient how to control heart palpitations with *auto-regulation* if he himself never learned to slow his own heart rate with *auto-regulation*.

How can I help her go limbic if I am so cortical myself?

Marty, a woman in her mid forties consulted me for nose and sinus allergy, heart palpitations, and episodes of dizziness and sweating. On two occasions, her coworkers had to call an ambulance to take her to the local hospital. After clinical evaluation and Micro-elisa blood tests for allergy caused by IgE type antibodies, I initiated our allergy and nutritional protocols.

I recognized that her cardiac symptoms were being induced by both allergic triggers and stress. Her cardiogram was normal. I knew we would not be able to completely control her palpitation attacks without eliminating her stress triggers. On a follow-up visit, I explained to her the need for self-regulation for controlling many of her symptoms. Also, I gave her an outline of my approach for this and my methods for *auto-reg*. She seemed to agree. So I took her to my *auto-reg* laboratory, attached to her body the appropriate electronic sensors, and started instruction. Within a few minutes, she suddenly seemed offended by what I was trying to do.

"I fear for my life. I am afraid I will collapse somewhere and die, and you act as if it is all in my head."

Marty spoke with evident anger.

My explanations seemed to feed her anger. Her words grew stronger. It was clear to me I was not going to succeed, and that I needed to somehow stop the session with whatever graces I could come up with. You cannot help everyone, I thought to myself. A few moments later I started to take the sensors off her skin. That is when I realized I was making the same mistake which I am always asking my patients to avoid. She was angry (and *cortical*). In my defense, I was also anxious and hurt (and *cortical*). How can I help her go *limbic* if I am so *cortical* myself?, I thought. There is no chance of success. But what would happen if I myself went *limbic*? The temptation was too great for me to resist.

I told Marty I was not going to charge her for this *auto-reg* laboratory session and asked her if she would do me a personal favor. Would she close her eyes, follow my words, and allow me to study her computer graphs for a few minutes. She was obviously opposed to it but somehow agreed. I started *Limbic Breathing* and momentarily slipped out of my *Cortical mode*. After some minutes, I opened my eyes and looked at the computer screen. Marty taught me an essential lesson.

Marty's biologic profile on the computer screen showed a sudden "melt-down". Melt-down is a term I use when I see a biologic profile abruptly change from a pattern of turbulence and stress (tall and sudden spikes like New York city skyline) to one of a calm, steady-state biology (smooth and even curves like the Kansas prairie). I froze the computer screen. I asked Marty to open her eyes and thanked her for those few moments. Marty seemed puzzled.

"I had bad cramps in my stomach. Now they are gone", she said. "What happened?"

I gave Marty a brief explanation of what had happened. Marty was now ready for *auto-reg*. She stayed with me in the laboratory for about thirty more minutes. She insisted on making payment for that *auto-reg* session. Several weeks later, she told me she felt "over 80% better". She became a regular *auto-regger*. During a recent visit (about 30 months after I first saw her), she said, "There is no problem now. I can control my heart palpitations and panic attacks with confidence."

SIXTH LESSON:
Medical technology has made surgery safe for the patient; the challenge now is to make the patient safe from surgery. Medical chemistry has made drugs potent; the challenge now is to make people safe from drug toxicity.

The problem of safe surgery is this: It obliterates the difference between the price paid for needed and un-needed surgery. It makes it difficult both for the surgeon and the patient to resist the temptation of a "quick fix" with a surgical strike when that is not the right way.

Historically, the balance in surgery was assured by the possibility of a fatal outcome. The surgeon knew this. A surgeon had to consider this, if for no other reason than to protect his reputation (and livelihood). The patient also knew this. That gave patient an additional level of safety.

The surgeon, however, should leave the sick man alone rather than operate, if he is in any doubt: for it is safer to leave a man in the hands of his creator, than to put trust in surgery or medicine concerning which there is any manner of doubt.

John Mirfield, 1362-1407

When in doubt, cut it out.

A surgical resident's cliche

Consider surgery which is pervasive today: gastrectomy for stomach ulcer, hysterectomy for pain, bowel surgery for colitis, excision of nerves (sympathectomy) for tight arteries, and TMJ surgery for jaw muscle spasms. This is the beginning of a long list of illnesses for which surgery is often readily performed. But these are states in which the patient should first give a fair chance to self-healing with self-regulatory methods, under the watchful eyes of a supportive physician. My surgeon friends do not disagree with this. This evidently does not hold for surgery for cancer, trauma, and acute surgical emergencies where undue delay often poses a real threat to life.

From a societal perspective, a good long-term solution to this problem is a significant reduction in the number of positions in the surgical training programs.

A surgeon busy with needed surgery is the best protection against un-needed surgery for a patient.

Drugs numb us. Drugs dull our sensitivity to our biology. Drugs deafen us to the incessant calls for relief from our body organs in distress. Reversal of chronic illness does not call for symptom-suppressing drugs, it calls for recognition and removal of the cause. Patients intuitively know all this. They do not want their biologies invaded by drugs, if it can be helped.

Given a choice between self-healing (with a supportive physician) and drug therapy, most people will choose self-regulation and healing for a chronic disease.

Drugs save lives for acute life-threatening illnesses. Drugs, in general, only suppress the symptoms of chronic diseases. A surgeon's scalpel never heals. An internist's drug never heals. The drugs and the surgical knife do, however, remove impediments in the way of cells and tissues healing by their natural felicity. Auto-regulation assists tissue healing in precisely the same way.

First do no harm. This is the first principle of Auto-regulation. This is a point important enough to be reiterated several times. No disease must be allowed to progress while the patient learns the principles and methods of Auto-regulation. Appropriate standard treatment methods must be used during this time.

Patients in self-healing want to be in safe custody of a professional who know this.

SEVENTH LESSON:
Psycho-somatic and somato-psychic models of disease are artifacts of our thinking.

Diseases are burdens on biology. Psyche (mind) and soma (body) are inseparable parts of our biology. This debate between psycho-somatic and somato-psychic models of disease is futile. It generates much heat but creates no light. As we become more enlightened in our biologic perspectives, I believe, this debate will die out.

Advances in behavioral biology and experimental psychology are putting these two disciplines on a collision course. Neuroanatomists are mapping out the human brain by defining the neuro-transmitters pathways. They are creating what Bartley Hoebel of Princeton University calls "a new psychological taxonomy based on chemical neuroanatomy." We are witnessing the dawn of a new science: *the science of oneness of the body and mind.*

Stress is an integral part of our biology. Stress can trigger, mimic, or exaggerate almost all disease processes. In biology, the stress response is an essential element of an organism's physiology. We cannot live without this response any more than we can live without a heart beating in our chest, or a brain creating impulses in our skulls. The stress response is composed of an inter-related series of electro-magnetic and physico-chemical events. These events throw our whole biology into a more strained state. Our pain becomes more acute, our suffering more intense. Success in Auto-regulation requires that we begin with success in stress control.

Focus on the biologic aspects of stress, and not the analysis of its causes, is a superior strategy when we are under stress.

Knowledge of the causes of stress is essential for prevention of stress. But this knowledge, by itself, cannot dissipate stress for us. Focus on the biologic consequences of the stress response (the condition of heart, brain and other body functions) gives far superior clinical benefits than any emphasis on the analysis of its causes. Specifically, in the methods of *auto-regulation*, we focus on the state of various body organs to obtain more consistent and predictable control of stress.

The problem for people is not the absence of desire to control stress, it is not knowing *how* to do it. Telling a patient under stress to relax is akin to telling a patient with a migraine attack to dissolve his headache without drug. If he could do so, he would not be suffering the way he is. For most patients in the throes of chronic illness and unremitting stress, the word "relax" does not carry any images for control of the biologic stress reactions.

By common life experience, we know what it means to be "relaxed", a state of physical and mental calm. By common experience, we also know that this alone does not help us in controlling stress.

The schematic diagram shown below outlines the principal psychophysiological inter-relationships of the stress response.

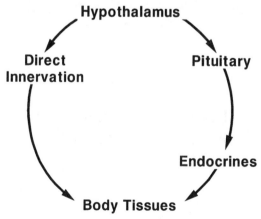

Stress Response

Hypothalamus

Direct Innervation

Pituitary

Endocrines

Body Tissues

Neutral And Endocrine Pathways

One essential aspect of stress which is often not fully recognized is that all the adverse effects of the stress response do not wear off soon after the stressor is removed. Indeed, in the diseases initiated, perpetuated, and worsened by stress, the intermediate and long-term effects of stress are much more important than the immediate effects.

The intermediate and long-term effects of the stress response are the root causes of many of the diseases of our time. Stress response puts our whole biology in a high gear, a state of *biologic burn-out*. What we call stress in common language is a highly complex and delicately balanced series of electro-magnetic and bio-chemical events. It causes anxiety, rapid heart rate, heart palpitations, sweating, abdominal cramps, diarrhea, muscle spasms, high blood pressure, spastic colitis, and eventually leads to chronic fatigue syndrome, stomach ulcers, heart disease and a host of other disorders.

EIGHTH LESSON:
The syndrome of our times is "The Dis-ease Syndrome"

The Dis-ease Syndrome is the pervasive clinical disorder of our times. It affects people of all ages, from our children to our senior citizens.

The Dis-ease Syndrome is a syndrome of a multitude of symptoms, a multitude of negative laboratory tests, a multitude of diagnostic labels, a multitude of prescriptions, and a deeply troubled patients.

> *The Dis-ease Syndrome is caused by the three major maladies of our times: stress, faulty nutrition, and sensitivity to environmental agents.*

Diseases, with some exceptions, are not sudden departures from health. Acute diseases, in general, are but the consequences of long-neglected *Dis-ease Syndrome.*

The benefits of science and technology are clear to all of us. Conquest of infectious diseases and safe surgery are crowning victories of modern medicine. But the threats to our health and survival unleashed by science and technology are often not as clear.

Life for most people has become a steady strife: before our biology can switch off its response to one stressor, it is confronted by another. Unrelenting stress is a relentless threat to our biology.

Our nutrition is in double jeopardy: our food is often depleted of essential micro-nutrients; and our biology is challenged with chemicals in preservatives, herbicides and pesticides with each meal.

Why do we develop and use pesticides and
herbicides? Obviously, it is to kill life.
Why do we add preservatives to our foods?
Obviously, it is to make food unsuitable
for consumption by other life forms.

It was our belief that we can kill life around us with these materials, but our molecules, cells, and tissues will not be effected by their adverse effects. We know better now. Pesticides (organophospates and organochlorides) kill insects by poisoning their enzymes (choline esterases). Recent studies have documented that these pesticides poison the same enzymes in the human immune cells as well.We have abraded and abused our habitat. Changes in our environments are sweeping in breadth and devastating in speed. We, as a species, cannot adapt to these changes with equal speed.

The diseases which afflict us are changing: so must our ideas of preventing and treating them.

*Everywhere the old order changes and
happy they who can change.*

Sir William Osler,M.D.

I have discussed the concepts of burdens on our biology,
the barometer of biology and The Dis-ease Syndrome in the
companion volume *The Dog and the Dis-ease Syndrome.*

NINTH LESSON:

**The primary determinant of disease prognosis,
with some exceptions, is the power of the mind.**

In the usual mode of medical practice, a patient's own
healing power is generally excluded from all deliberations
concerning the diagnosis, treatment, and prognosis of his
disease process,

The diagnosis is made by history, clinical examination,

laboratory tests, X-rays, and, on many occasions, a biopsy of the organ involved.

The prognosis comes straight out of the statistics in medical texts. These statistics are derived from studies conducted with treatment modalities under "double-blind, cross-over" conditions. The term "double-blind" means that neither the patient nor the physician knows whether the treatment consists of a drug or a placebo (starch pill). The term "cross-over" means that the order of the use of the drug and the placebo is reversed in the second part of the trial. This method is rightfully considered as the most objective method for assessing the efficacy of new drugs.

The essential weakness of the double-blind cross-over method is this: it blinds the patient to the mode of treatment used, and by definition, excludes him from any role that he may play in his recovery from disease.

Why do we so emphatically, and dogmatically, exclude the healing power of the patient from our treatment strategies? The answer is quite simple. Because historically we could not measure and quantify this power. Since it could not be measured, it was denied. But must we continue to do so for ever? Is it still not possible to design methods for measuring this power of healing in objective ways? Of course it can be. Should we, then, not design new treatment strategies to fully benefit from this greatest of all healing resources? Of course we should. This is the essence of Auto-regulation.

This essential concept of the healing power of the patient can be best illustrated with a commonly encountered clinical problem.

A business executive in his mid-forties is found to have hypertension (high blood pressure). His physician orders various tests to find the cause of his hypertension. All tests results are negative. The physician makes the diagnosis of essential hypertension (the type of hypertension which is generally believed to be of unknown cause). The physician gives his patient the prognosis for hypertension given in medical texts. Hypertension causes damage to heart, arteries, kidneys and brain. Untreated, it will eventually will cause heart failure, and may lead to other serious complications such as stroke and kidney failure.

Next, the physician prescribes one or more drugs, to be taken for the rest of the patient's life (again according to the prevailing medical standards). This scenario is played out in this country a million times a year.

Loosening up the tight arteries.

Now let us consider the case history of Mary, and the

results of an self-regulatory approach. Mary, a single parent in her thirties, consulted us for hypertension with a blood pressure of 230/130. A diagnosis of essential hypertension had been made previously. She had been prescribed a variety of drugs to lower her blood pressure. She was unable to take these drugs for any length of time due to side-effects.

After a complete clinical evaluation, I explained to Mary that her blood pressure was high because her arteries were tight (in a state of spasm). Further, I explained that her arteries were held tight by her biology responding to some stressors in her life. We discussed how some stressors in her life situations might be avoided. I also prescribed one of the anti-hypertensive drugs in a small dose.

Next, I gave her instruction in the principles and methods of *auto-regulation*. As she became proficient in the practice of *auto-regulation*, I gradually reduced the dose of her medicine. Ten weeks later, Mary normalized her blood pressure down to a healthy level of 130/80 without taking any drugs. Mary also gained important insight into the cumulative adverse impact of the stressors in her life on her biology.

Is this case history fictional? A delusional plausibility of an idealogue? Was Mary playing some sordid trick? Taking drugs for lowering blood pressure without telling me? I do not believe so. I have observed this phenomenon too many times to doubt Mary's veracity.

Can most diseases be approached in this fashion? The answer is an unequivocal "yes". Will success with *auto-regulation* be so dramatic in all cases? Probably not. Some benefits of auto-regulation, however, are evident to everybody who persists even with his work with these methods, even for a few weeks.

Sir William Osler, M.D., probably the best-known physician of the early part of this century, believed that the prognosis of a patient with tuberculosis of the lung depends less on what is in his lungs and more on what is in his head. Sir Osler is not alone in his thinking. Thinkers in medicine of all ages eventually arrived at varying notions of the same fundamental themes.

TENTH LESSON:

The issues of the placebo effect, false hope, guilt of failure, and "the Exceptional Patient Syndrome" are not essential issues for the patients in self-regulation and healing.

Different diseases afflict people in different ways. Diseases cause pain and suffering in different ways, and for different lengths of time. Some diseases can be cured with self-regulation in a few weeks. Some call for months of training and practice. Some indeed require a life-long commitment.

Drugs can be avoided altogether for many diseases. Drug use can be drastically reduced in many other diseases. Drug use can be limited to only true emergencies for yet other disorders.

Patients learn all this well. They value all such understanding. Even in instances when unremitting suffering from a chronic refractory illness blocked progress in *auto-regulation*, my patients were still grateful for the hope that one day they will move ahead with self-healing.

Professionals often express deep concerns about the problems which may arise from the issues of the placebo effect, false hope, guilt of failure, and the "Exceptional Patient syndrome". I do not see any patients who want, or even care to, discuss these issues. Patients want relief of symptoms. They want freedom from pain and disease. They want their health restored. Self-regulation, of course, means regulating one's own biology. They do not have any difficulty in understanding the principles and practice of self-regulation.

If the patients do not care for these issues, why do we professionals do so? It puzzles me. I suppose these problems arise from mis-communications and misunderstandings between the patient and the professional. I have discussed these issues in greater detail in the section on *Placebo-busters, Placebo-phobes, and Placebo-philes* in the companion volume *The Pheasant and Suffering in Illness.*

Lessons learned
from patients with cancer

Life is a gift. It should be treasured above all other gifts one receives.

Life is a terminal condition. None of us is going to get out of it.

There is no point in preparing for death. The only preparation one needs to make is to live the *present* moment.

Prognosis in cancer depends upon two elements: the biology of the tumor and the biology of the person. Cancer survival figures are not relevant to an individual patient with cancer. A patient with cancer must find the professional with necessary expertise who confronts the biology of the tumor; he alone can sustain his own biology.

Suffering for patients with cancer has three faces: a face of the suffering of the *moment*, a face of remembered suffering, and a face of feared future suffering.

What is the reality of life? That single moment of the

present. Hope, despair, love and hatred are all events which make up the *present* moment. These are all electro-magnetic and biochemical events which determine the state of the human condition, which, in turn, affects the way our biology copes with the burdens of cancer, and wins or loses. We may see and live our lives in the *present* moment, or may live with remembered suffering or feared future suffering. All our memories of the past flow from the *present* as do all fears (and hopes) for the future.

The pain and suffering in any single moment of the *present* is no greater for a person if he were to live for one more year, and it is no lesser if he were to live for thirty more years.

How does a patient with cancer learn to live in the *present moment* as if it were the last moment of life? Through anguish and suffering, and through knowledge and love. Many patients seem to intuitively learn this; some others learn through love and compassion of others. There are still others who never do, often because they are not aware of this possibility (or deny it). Those who do learn often find totally unexpected rewards: love finds a new expression when it emanates from living in the *moment.*

My surgeon-friends who have done a lot of cancer surgery agree with this: patients who learn to live in the *moment* live fuller and longer lives.

Section 3

The Elephant and Star Wars Medicine

*The quality of medical care is an
index of civilization.*

Committee on Costs of Medical care, 1932

*Today "care" is no longer enough; patients now
expect, and physicians try very hard for, "cure", often to
the detriment of caring as it was known in the 1930s
and 1940s.*

Annals of Internal Medicine
Editorial, 12:637, 1990

Three Miracles of Modern Medicine

The thought of "Star Wars Medicine" crossed my mind one
day recently as I sat in Marian hall at Holy Name Hospital,
Teaneck, N.J. Three cases of cardiac tamponade, all young

patients brought to the hospital in a near-death condition, were presented in this conference. Cardiac tamponade is a life-threatening condition in which the heart muscle is fatally compressed by blood or fluid rapidly collecting within the pericardium, the thick sheath of tissue which encases the heart. The heart is literally choked to death.

TAMPONADE CAUSED BY A RUPTURED AORTA

The first patient collapsed at home and was rushed to the emergency department with a dissecting aortic aneurysm. She had spontaneously ruptured her aorta into her pericardium. The aorta is the main arterial trunk which carries blood from the heart. The pericardium fills up with blood rapidly when the aorta ruptures into it. This catastrophe is uniformly fatal if not diagnosed and corrected immediately.

Her physicians made the diagnosis of a ruptured aorta promptly by putting a large needle into the pericardium. She was rushed to the operating room. Her aorta was cut across, the tear in the wall of the aorta was sutured, and the repaired aorta was sutured back to the heart. The wall of the aorta in a case of aneurysm is thinned out, frayed, and friable. This makes such an operation far more complex and technically demanding than a heart transplant. She recovered and went home.

Now the medical staff of Holy Name Hospital sat in the conference hall watching on a video screen the movements of a choked heart, the outline of its chambers, and the flow of blood through the torn wall of the aorta. The physician audience was visibly moved by this true-to-life, vivid, dramatic and futuristic sight. They knew that a torn aorta had been an unforgiving killer in our hospital until recently.

TAMPONADE CAUSED BY A VIRAL INFECTION

The second patient collapsed at home with chest pain. She was rushed to the emergency department, again in a near-death condition. Her physicians suspected cardiac tamponade from physical examination. Rapid accumulation of fluid caused by a viral infection of the pericardium was choking her heart. Her life was in an immediate danger. There was no room for diagnostic error or delay if she was to have any chance for survival.

The staff of the emergency department learned from her family that she had been in excellent health until a few days earlier when she developed a respiratory viral infection. Again, her attending physicians made a prompt diagnosis with an exploratory needle. She was rushed to the operating room. Her surgeon cut a window in her pericardium to let the fluid drain out. She made an uneventful recovery. Again, the physician audience was demonstrably impressed by the speed, accuracy and efficiency of her team of doctors and nurses.

TAMPONADE CAUSED BY LUPUS

The third patient was rushed to the hospital with a cardiac tamponade which occurred as a complication of systemic lupus. Her diagnosis, suspected from clinical examination, was quickly established with an exploratory needle. Her situation improved dramatically with simple aspiration of the fluid collection within her pericardium. She went home without any surgery. For the third time, the physician audience looked impressed. All of us physicians had too many memories of patients lost to such devastating accidents of biology to take things for granted.

Star War Medicine! That is the only way I could see all this. A mere three decades earlier, as a medical student, I had committed to memory the names of these diseases among a list of sure killers. Now it all seemed simple and straight forward. Three patients in moribund condition. Three teams of doctors and nurses. Three successful therapeutic strategies. Three cases presented as mere mechanical problems; a string of events which made the improbable seem so utterly routine.

I marveled at these astounding feats of precision in diagnosis and promptness in treatment of these sure-killers of yester-year.

Some hours later, I went to the hospital library looking for some references. I chanced upon a recent issue of the *Annals of Internal Medicine* which carried a position paper prepared by the American College of Physicians. It began,

"The American College of Physicians believes that there is an increasingly urgent need to address a growing problem, that of many Americans lacking access to health care........ Total health care expenditure have risen from $ 75 billions in 1970 to approximately $ 600 billions in 1989......"

Twenty pages later, the position paper concluded,

"The American College of Physicians believes that it is time to confront the issue of access to health care. Piecemeal solutions to a national problem of this magnitude will not suffice...... Reliance solely on private charity or the efforts of individual states--with differing

*and variable resources--to assure that the national need
is met is a fundamental abrogation of this overreaching
responsibility....."*

Annals of Internal Medicine
112:641-661, 1990.

In this lengthy position paper, the College did not deem it
necessary to discuss the enormous potential of preventive
medicine for reducing the cost of medical care (and increasing
access to care).

Beyond disease prevention, there are the possibilities of
disease treatment with nutritional medicine, environmental
medicine, medicine of self-regulation and the medicine of
fitness. I wrote in the preface of this book that I regard these
medical disciplines as the four faces of a new approach to
molecular medicine. The cost of disease reversal with the
treatment protocols of molecular medicine in most instances is
substantially lower than that with the classical approach with
drugs.

I do not agree with the position taken by the American
College of Physicians about what constitutes *a fundamental
abrogation of this overreaching responsibility.* I look at the issue
of access to care in a different light. The real problem, in my
judgement, is our preoccupation with the glamour of the Star
Wars Medicine which is robbing us of common sense in
medicine. Not offering patients in the throes of chronic illness
effective treatment protocols of molecular medicine, is, in my

judgement, *a fundamental abrogation of this overreaching responsibility.*

How many do not need Star Wars Medicine ?

Stress, obesity, smoking, caffeinism, alcoholic tissue injury and substance abuse. These are the major threats to health. Star Wars Medicine has little to offer for any of them.

Hypertension (high blood pressure) may occur in as many as 58 million Americans (Arch. Intern. Med. 148:1023-38, 1988). Do these people need the Star Wars Medicine?

With rare exceptions, individuals with hypertension do not need the high-tech Star Wars Medicine. They need to learn how to listen to their tissues, open up their arteries, and normalize their blood pressure. High blood pressure is caused by tight arteries. Arteries tighten up in response to burdens on biology: burdens of stress, of functional nutritional deficiencies, of environmental triggers, of lack of physical fitness, and of immune dysfunctions. Hypertension, first and foremost, calls for treatment protocols of molecular medicine (nutritional and environmental medicine, and medicine of self-regulation and fitness).

Coronary artery disease leads to 1.5 million heart attacks and over 500,000 deaths every year in America (American Heart Association. 1989 Heart Facts, Dallas, Texas.). Do these people need the Star Wars Medicine? Yes, they do, but only near the end.

Heart disease calls for Star Wars Medicine only after it has been neglected for years. A heart tires when it has to pump blood against tight arteries for years. A heart weakens if it is deprived of energy by plaque formation in its arteries (coronary arteriosclerosis). It quickens its rate, enlarges to cope with increased demands, and eventually fails. The prohibitively expensive technology of Star Wars Medicine is not required for dealing with the problems of a tired heart and clogged arteries. The low cost treatment protocols of molecular medicine are more effective measures for prolonging useful life. Coronary bypass surgery is done about six times as frequently in the U.S. as in England (Scientific American, July 1990). Extensive studies have been conducted at the Veterans Administration Hospital system comparing the benefits of heart surgery with conservative medical treatment for advanced coronary artery disease. Such studies fail to show any clear advantage of the surgical approach.

Stroke kills over 150,000 Americans every year. Do they need Star Wars Medicine? Yes, they do. But does Star Wars Medicine bring back to life their paralyzed limbs or restore their lost speech? The answer is a clear "No". With rare exceptions, strokes occur as complications of hypertension and plaque formation in arteries (arteriosclerosis). It calls for treatment of hypertension and arteriosclerosis with protocols of nutritional medicine and without the high-tech intervention of the Star Wars Medicine.

Cancer ranks third among the causes of death in the U.S.A. Do patients with cancer need Star War Medicine? They do, most assuredly, but even here, we choose to see only parts of the elephant (or are unable to see the whole elephant).

Our "war on cancer" is laughable.

Cancer begins as a damaged cell. The initial event in cell damage is molecular injury to the cell DNA. This is where we can hope to make the most difference, and this is where we fail. The DNA in each cell is being constantly injured and repaired; the injury is caused by free radicals (unbalanced high energy molecules which behave erratically), and it is repaired by cell enzymes called synthetases.

Excess free radicals are generated by stress, environmental pollutants, drugs, chemicals, radiation, and infection by microbes. Nature has provided us with the means to neutralize these radicals. Nutrients of major importance in this context are vitamins C and E, glutathione, taurine, cysteine, and many others. Their are still other ways excess free radicals can be quenched by appropriate protocols of molecular medicine.

It has been clear for quite some time that our *war on cancer* is misdirected. There is a great potential for prevention of cancer if we direct our resources and energy to the initial electro-magnetic and molecular event which initiate the DNA injury and lead to cancer. We choose to ignore this altogether. We are very vocal about eating oat bran (thanks largely to commercials of oat bran vendors), but that is about as far as our *war on cancer* goes. We spend billions of dollars on chemotherapy, radiotherapy, and extensive surgery for patients with advanced disseminated cancers. We totally ignore the roles that nutritional medicine, environmental medicine, and medicine of self-regulation can play in our *war against cancer.*

Our surgeons do excellent work whenever they do get a crack at a curative strike for early cancer. Unfortunately, this is not possible for a majority of patients with cancer.

"... we are losing the war against cancer, notwithstanding progress against several uncommon forms of the disease, improvements in palliation, and extension of the productive years of life. A shift in research emphasis, from research on treatment to research on prevention, seems necessary if substantial progress against cancer is to be forthcoming."

New England Journal of Medicine
1986; 314:1226-32

Very few of us look at the whole elephant of cancer. By and large, we ignore the larger issues in causation of cancer. Our *war on cancer* is laughable. Could it be that there is indeed a grand design (which some claim exists but of which I am not aware) to focus our energies on smaller issues of one or the other regimens of chemotherapy or radiotherapy, and ignore the larger issues of enhancing those immune functions which the body uses to ward off mutant cancer cells with damaged DNA. Consider the following excerpt.

Cancers of colon, breast, and prostate, the three forms of cancer most closely associated epidemiologically with nutritional factors, together cause over 130,000 deaths.

> Guide to Clinical Preventive Services, Report of the US Preventive Services Task Force, 1989.

Medical opinions such as the one expressed above are singularly devoid of any value, both for the physician and for the patient. All cancers are the result of the impact of nutritional and environments triggers on the genetic make-up if we consider this issue in broader terms of the true molecular nature and cause of cancer. I wonder if there has ever been a single patient who was saved from a cancer or a single physician who treated a cancer more effectively just because he knew that this Task Force thinks cancers of colon, breast and prostate cancers are epidemiologically associated with nutritional factors.

Hurt caused by Star Wars Medicine

Star Wars Medicine saves many lives. It extends productive lives of millions of others. I see miracles of Star Wars Medicine every day. I see these miracles in the operating rooms, intensive care units, emergency departments, and other wards of Holy Name and other hospitals. I have had the privilege of being a part of the teams of physicians, nurses, and other hospital staff who served as the instruments of such miracles for over quarter of a century.

The benefits of Star Wars Medicine are well-recognized. What is not equally well-recognized is how many are hurt, often severely, by this type of medicine. For many patients, Star Wars Medicine strives to close the proverbial barn door a little too late for the patient.

Every day I also see the hurt caused by this Star Wars Medicine. How does Star Wars Medicine hurt?

BRIDGETTE'S STORY

Bridgette, a French woman in her late thirties, moved to

the U.S. in the mid-1980s when her husband moved his business from Europe to this country. Within several months, she developed dizzy spells and chest spasms. Her symptoms progressed and became incapacitating. She was forced to give up driving. One morning she woke up and found herself unable to move her limbs. Karen's husband, Pierre, was away in Europe on a business trip. A neighbor called an ambulance and agreed to care for her three year old son.

She stayed in the hospital for over two weeks. She was examined by several specialists and underwent exhaustive diagnostic tests including multiple CAT scans and cardiac evaluation with an Holter monitor. Her physicians were very supportive. While in the hospital, she received multiple drug therapies. She was discharged from the hospital without a diagnosis and with nine different prescriptions for various medications. Some months later Bridgette and Pierre returned to Europe.

During our recent trip to Europe, Pierre and Bridgette invited Talat and me for dinner. Bridgette felt she had almost completely recovered from her *illness*. It took patience and persistent efforts on her part to gradually wean herself from all the drugs she had been put on after her hospitalization in the U.S. Her physician in Europe had been very supportive. She was still unable to drive for fear of dizzy spells.

Looking back at her illness now, after some years, she thought she knew what had ailed her then. She felt strongly that she neither needed nor benefitted from the high tech tools of Star Wars medicine with which she was treated during her hospital stay. The causes of her illness were quite apparent to her. She had been alone with a small child for weeks when her husband was away on business trips. There were no Europeans in her community. There were frequent reports of mugging and other crimes in her town. She became extremely concerned about her safety. Installation of an alarm system seemed to only feed upon her fears. Then came the news of a violent break-in her neighborhood. Fear and anxiety evolved into episodes of chest pain, palpitations, and dizziness. The last straw turned out to be the paralyzing panic attack that morning of hospitalization.

Bridgette felt sure of the true nature of her illness. For one thing, Star Wars Medicine in the U.S. had failed to establish her *diagnosis*. For another, her illness cleared up without additional treatment on her return to Europe.

Next, she told us with evident bitterness in her voice how her family was still making monthly payments after some years of that illness toward the huge hospital bill.

Is Bridgette an exceptional case? What American physician with any length of clinical experience would regard this case history as unusual? At present, about forty million Americans do not have any medical insurance. Star Wars Medicine punishes, financially and emotionally, hundreds of thousands of people like Bridgette every year. They have procedures done to them which can be avoided. They are required to pay for services which are unnecessary.

Star Wars Hospitalopathy

I use the term "Star Wars Hospital-opathy" to refer to a variety of pathologic states created by Star Wars Medicine, usually but not always in hospitalized patients. It is a growing menace. It is simplistic to look for the villains in this sad story among any group of health professionals or among patients or in our judicial system. It is the nature of the beast.

Access to Star Wars technology without clinical and philosophical maturity is like political freedom without a civic sense of responsibility.

A society cannot ask for one without the other. The mechanics of Star Wars Medicine must be subordinated to common sense in looking at the molecular menagerie of human biology.

BILL'S STORY

Bill, a man in his late sixties, drove to the hospital for a bronchoscopy and some other diagnostic tests. He suffered from chronic cough and had coughed up some blood. He had a lung cancer removed four years earlier. Since then he had remained free of cancer. Bill had smoked for years and had developed emphysema of the lung. Bronchoscopy was now planned to rule out the possibility of recurrent cancer.

Bronchoscopy and lung biopsy procedure went well. Fortunately, the lung biopsy proved to be negative, and so did several sputum examinations, CAT scan and several other tests. The lung biopsy showed some inflammation of the lung, and he was prescribed antibiotics. His physician was still very concerned about the possibility of recurrence of a tumor.

During the next four weeks, Bill received different antibiotics, multiple drugs for cough, shortness of breath, high blood pressure, anxiety and poor sleep. His general condition continued to deteriorate. He grew progressively weak and developed a variety of symptoms. Many sophisticated computerized lung function and blood gas tests were performed. He was seen by several consultants. After each visit by a different physician, he asked about his diagnosis. None was forthcoming. He became depressed. More tests followed more drugs. More drugs caused adverse effects and required yet more drugs to control these effects. *Star Wars Medicine was in full swing.*

Bill became convinced that his physicians and his family were withholding information from him. He became increasingly anxious, distraught and depressed. One day I went to see him. I had known Bill for several years. He knew I had examined his lung biopsy and reviewed the results of other tests. He asked me, as he had asked on other occasions, if I knew what his diagnosis was. I told him his lung biopsy showed mild interstitial pneumonitis, a type of lung inflammation which is usually caused by viral infections and which sometimes takes weeks to clear up. The biopsy and all other tests were negative for cancer. Her wanted to know if that was all there was to know. Why were so many different physicians called upon to see him and why couldn't they give him a diagnosis. I tried to explain further. He listened to my explanation with eyes full of disappointment.

Bill had good reason for his disappointment. I did not say what I really wanted to say. I wanted to tell him that life is a terminal condition, and that none of us can avoid death. I wanted to say that the risk of cancer recurrence for him was there, and, that to the best of our knowledge, he was free of cancer at this time. I wanted him to know that what ailed him now was "Star Wars Hospitalopathy". This is a disorder for which we have no drugs. Our Star Wars machines are totally helpless against this fell disorder. It is a disorder seen in hospitalized patients in which there is a "molecular burn-out", a pattern of injury to molecules caused by free radicals. Free radicals are very small, highly unstable and noxious molecules which are produced by some larger molecules generated by stress, fear, and despair. Free radicals are produced by the physical invasion of body tissues with tubes, catheters and other instruments. Drugs become free radicals as the body tries to rid itself of them. Drugs also produce free radicals by blocking normal molecular pathways. Degenerative disorders, metabolic disorders, infections, radiation, all cause excessive production of free radicals.

I wanted to tell him that Star Wars Medicine had cleared him of definable cancer, but it had also injured his molecules and cells. I wanted to tell him to go home so his injured molecules and cells can have a chance to recover. But I could not say it. The diagnosis of *Star Wars Hospitalopathy* was real but modern medicine had yet not proven this with its *blessed* double-blind cross-over model of research, and that it had not yet been accepted as a part of our *blessed* prevailing standards of care. So I kept quiet. It would not have been so bad if Bill was not been such a perceptive individual. He knew something deeply troubled me. He must have thought it was the diagnosis of cancer which I was keeping from him.

The proper management of *Star Wars Hospitalopathy* requires that the patient be taken out of the environments which make him sick. It requires that we teach him how to lower his "molecular thermostat" with methods of self-regulation. Finally, it requires that we support him with appropriate protocols of nutritional medicine. In short, it calls for the non-drug, non-interventionist protocols of molecular medicine.

I could not say all this to Bill. It will be a long time before *Star Wars Hospitalopathy* becomes a *scientifically* acceptable medical diagnosis.

High blood pressure had not been a major problem for Bill. But that was before he was hospitalized. Now his days were full of despair and his nights filled with panic. Bill developed a stroke and lost the use of one arm and one leg. A decision was made to refer Bill to another institution for rehabilitation.

A week later, Bill's son spoke of his sadness,

"It wouldn't be so sad if he did not know that he is being passed up as a lost cause. He overheard someone say that severely debilitated cases like him are usually not accepted by that hospital for active rehab work. This is a man who was hanging curtains two days before he walked into this hospital, and now he is considered unfit for transfer to a rehab place."

Star Wars Medicine hurts in many ways.

THE DIS-EASE SYNDROME

There is a new epidemic among people who are "not

healthy". The technology of Star Wars Medicine cannot quantify the state of being "not healthy". Medical texts have no descriptions of this syndrome. It is a syndrome of *molecular injury and immune dysfunction* caused by the stress of modern (speeded-up) life, poor nutrition, vulnerability to environments, and lack of physical fitness. Viral and other infections follow as the molecular and immune defenses falter. I call this "The Dis-ease Syndrome".

The Dis-ease Syndrome affects different people in different ways. There is one common thread: all individuals with this syndrome know they are not healthy. They have had many laboratory tests with negative results. They know they are under stress, suffer from frequent infections, and eat poorly. However, rarely do they recognize the degree of their molecular injury and the depth of their immune dysregulation.

The symptoms of *The Dis-ease Syndrome* are many and varied. Vague and hard-to-define symptoms include undue lassitude, mid-morning tiredness, lack of vigor, and a sense of being "drained". Subjective symptoms of anxiety, jitteryness, unexplained mood swings, inability to concentrate, and short attention span occur often.

Stiffness in joints, sometimes with swelling, occur more often in young women. Chronic headache, pressure in sinus areas, tension in neck and back muscles, and muscle spasm are experienced commonly by both women and men. Other symptoms include tightness in chest, palpitations, indigestion, abdominal bloating and cramps, burning "in the pit of stomach", and episodes of diarrhea. In young women, the incidence of incapacitating premenstrual syndrome is high.

Most importantly, *the Dis-ease Syndrome* manifests itself as recurrent infections. Such individuals go from one infection to another with repeated courses of antibiotics, often with severe damage to their bowel ecology and resulting yeast infections. The infections appear as sore throats, tonsillitis, ear infections, upper respiratory "viral" infections, cystitis and urinary tract infections and vaginitis. At other times, *the Dis-ease Syndrome* first presents itself with specific infections such as herpes blisters, Epstein-Barre virus infection, cytomegalic virus infection, toxoplasmosis and infections caused by a host of other microbes.

Regional infections often draw the attention away from the real issues of antecedent molecular injury and immune dysregulation. Antibiotic therapy, of course, provides temporary control of bacterial infections, and sets the patient up for still more molecular and immune injury.

"This kid comes in with cramps and some blood in stools. His colon biopsy shows mild non-specific inflammation. I put him on antibiotics. He is not getting better. There is this thing about mother nature. People either get better or worse. I am going to switch the antibiotics. We will see."

Overheard.

Yes, there is this thing about mother nature. It does know

how to repair injured molecules. It does it so very well. But antibiotics do not make it easier for mother nature. Antibiotics kill life, *bad* forms of life as well as good forms of life. The bowel ecology is damaged by antibiotics. One accepts this damage only if the risk of infections is clear and immediate and if one has a broader game plan to manage the MIS Syndrome with appropriate non-drug protocols of molecular medicine.

Star Wars Medicine hurts people with *the Dis-ease Syndrome. It does so* in two ways.

First,

The tools of this medicine further increase their suffering by imposing new burdens on their biology.

Second,

It withholds from them the treatment protocols of molecular medicine which are designed to eliminate or reduce the various burdens which *The Dis-ease Syndrome* imposes upon their biology.

I have discussed the known essentials of the basic chemistry of life, free radical production in tissues, molecular injury caused by free radicals, our increasing sensitivity to environmental pollutants, development of insidious and persistent immune dysfunctions, and, finally, the full clinical expression of *the Dis-ease Syndrome* in the companion volume *The Dog and the Dis-ease Syndrome.*

TUSKS, TRUNK, TORSO, OR TAIL
OF THE ELEPHANT

How did we physicians get committed to the theme of *testing and treating only parts of our patients*?   How did the healing arts evolve into a medicine which looks at bits and fragments of a sick person, and devises treatment strategies as if the person attached to that bit of tissue is irrelevant to the process of healing?

How did we physicians become subservient to the theme of chemical solutions to all our health problems?

Why is nutritional medicine so misunderstood?   Why is environmental medicine so maligned? Why is the medicine of self-regulation so often dismissed as *fringe medicine?*

How did we physicians get caught up in a medicine which *treats* mere *diagnostic labels* as it professes to *care* for the sick people?

How did we physicians get trapped in a system which defies common sense? How did we physicians get so confused about what constitutes *caring* and what constitutes *curing?*

Why do we ignore the larger issues of the full impact of all the burdens on an individual's biology? Why do we choose to palpate, auscultate, or sense electronically, only small portions of the bodies of our patients? Why do we choose to see only the tusks, trunk, torso, or tail of the elephant?

These are the real issues facing medicine today. These are the issues which the American College of Physicians chose to ignore completely in their recent position paper.

I addressed these most fundamental of all questions facing medicine in my book *Nutritional Medicine: Principles and Practice.* I reproduce below some text from that volume:

Perfection of means and confusion of goals seem -- in my opinion -- to characterize our age.

AlbertEinstein

In *acute illness,* our *perfection of means* is astounding. Advances in medical technology are breathtaking. Our surgical prowess is daunting; the potency of our drugs limitless.

In *chronic illness,* our *confusion of goals* is equally astounding. We seem to think nutritional medicine is a hoax; environmental medicine, a treatment of non-existent disease; and self-healing, a wishful and simple-minded pursuit.

We seem to think that molecular and electro-magnetic events which initiate disease, and cell membrane dynamics which perpetuate it, are of little relevance to *clinical medicine.* We seem to think that to name a disease is to understand it; to classify it is to conquer it; to suppress its symptoms with drugs is to cure it.

Our principal strategy seems to be this: *disease prevention* is a patient's responsibility; when a patient is acutely ill, we pull him out of the jaws of death with miracles of modern medicine.

How could we, the healing profession, be so wrong?

Treating a disease is not the same thing as treating a patient.

Medicine started out as a calling. It turned into a profession. Then, it evolved into an industry. Now it has become big business.

The business of medicine is procedure-oriented. It has carved out for itself an area of rich profitability: the procedures, and the numbers these procedures produce for the acutely ill. This is easy to see because that is where the money in medicine is. We pay well for procedures and numbers (even when we know the procedures are unnecessary and the numbers worthless); we punish non-invasive protocols for treatment, by default if not by design. The business of medicine is not interested in disease prevention. This is easy to see as well. There is no money in disease prevention.

When medicine was a profession, the physician had both freedom and responsibility. His responsibility was to listen to the patient, seek out what made the patient sick, help reverse his illness, and teach him how to prevent recurrence of that disease. He had the freedom to practice medicine, unburdened by the demands of any third party payers.

Sanitation, vaccination, control of bacterial infections with antibiotics, and safe surgery brought forth the idea that medical technology could conquer all diseases, and that analytic technology could make all diagnoses.

The emergence of the health industry brought forth the idea that the cost of medicine could be obliterated, both for the patient and the physician. The patient could put his signature on some form, and the physician would be reimbursed by an agency. Thus, the physician became a provider, and the patient, a recipient of care. The *industry*, in the garb of a "thirdparty" payer, weakened the contract between the patient and the physician. Procedures became reimbursable services. *Listening to the patient became a non-reimbursable, and hence, an optional activity.*

When medicine became big business, requirements of momentum of the business called for more procedures, done more frequently and with increasing complexity. With fattening financial largess, it was predictable that scavengers will make the scene. The prey looked for a defense against the predator;

defensive medicine was born. Yet more procedures, more tests, more numbers, and more reasons for avoiding the labor of thinking.

The drug industry found its own opportunity in procedures and numbers. Anything which could not be supported by procedures and numbers was not worth an inquiry. This included that most valuable of all resources: a physician's clinical acumen.

Tyranny of numbers

Medicine became a numbers game. Initially, neither the physician nor the patient recognized the perils of numbers. Numbers in medicine came to determine the worth of a physician's work. Physicians who excelled at generating numbers were rewarded well. Those who didn't came to be regarded as lesser physicians. Early evolving disease produces no numbers. So it was ignored. Prevention of disease became non-reimbursable and, hence, optional.

Advanced disease produces many numbers, and so it became the *real* medicine. The stage was set for the tyranny of the numbers.

Bad numbers drove good sense out of our work as physician. Listening to the patient became redundant. When the numbers were *right,* the patient's suffering was recognized;

when they were not and the patient did not fit into our templates of disease, we dismissed him as a malingerer. When the numbers were *right*, the physician's work was honored; when they were not, the physician faced the indignity of being considered a *non-scientist*.

In our medical boards, we defended *the numbers* more fiercely than the Aztecs did their tribal Gods. Little did we realize that these numbers became our deities. We made many sacrifices at the alters of our *numerical Gods.*

A New Medicine

I see a new possibility of a molecular medicine: a medicine of molecules, of electron transfer, and of energy.

This new molecular medicine is applied physiology of fitness, applied pharmacology of nutrients, applied chemistry of environments, applied immunology of allergy, applied pathology of autoimmunity and applied biology of self-regulation. It is a medicine in which chronic disorders are treated without drugs; the treatment protocols are based on how molecules function in *health* rather than on how drugs suppress symptoms after cellular damage has been inflicted by *disease.*

This new medicine has four faces: nutritional medicine, environmental medicine, medicine of fitness, and medicine of self-regulation. What binds these four disciplines of molecular medicine together is molecular pathology. Perhaps it can be called "Clinical Molecology".

Nutritional medicine is a misunderstood Medicine.

Why is nutritional medicine so misunderstood by most physicians? There are several reasons for this.

First,

We physicians spend some hours in the study of the chemistry of nutrients in medical schools when our goals are passing grades. We spent a lifetime in clinical medicine devoted to the study of the chemistry of drugs. In classical clinical medicine, there is no need to think about the chemistry of nutrients. Why learn something we have no intentions of using?

Second,

We physicians are brought up with the notion that micro-nutrients are necessary for the prevention of *deficiency* syndromes (ascorbic acid for scurvy, niacin for pellagra, etc.) We generally have little or no appreciation of the *optimal metabolic requirements* of these nutrients in disease reversal and health preservation. The critical roles of essential fatty acids, minerals and other micro-nutrients are totally ignored in clinical medicine.

Third,

We physicians are brought up with concepts of cellular pathology. Our understanding of disease processes is based upon what we observe in cells with microscopes *after* the cells have been damaged. The rational practice of nutritional medicine can be based only upon the precepts of molecular pathology, a discipline in pathology which considers the molecular disarray which develops *before* molecular and cellular injury occurs.

Fourth,

We physicians are brought up to be interventionists. We learn to use drugs to "stamp out disease", with speed and efficiency. Drugs act by blocking, inhibiting or impairing in other ways the various electro-magnetic, molecular, and enzymatic processes in our biology. Our *drug of choice* is ideally a single agent which is intended to realize these goals.

Nutritional medicine, by contrast, calls for a restorative orientation. The strategy in nutritional medicine is not prompt intervention and expeditious interruption of molecular events. Rather, it is to provide a large array of nutrient molecules in optimal proportions to replenish a host of molecular pathways.

Where drugs act rapidly, nutrients deliver their benefits slowly. Interventionists that we are, drugs are a bigger draw for us.

Fifth,

We physicians are brought up with the dogma of the three D s: we are taught to think of one *disease*, make one *diagnosis*, and prescribe one *drug* of choice.

The dogma of the three D s served us well when our enemies were specific infections such as tuberculosis, leprosy and syphilis. The search for one disease, formulation of one diagnosis, and use of one drug allowed us to effectively eradicate a specific infection. Our conquest of infectious disease has been a crowning victory of modern medicine.

Times have changed. Our diseases have changed. The dominant chronic disorders of our time are problems of stress, nutrition, fitness, sensitivity to environmental agents, and immune dysfunctions caused by viral infections. These disorders feed upon each other. The precepts of the dogma of the three Ds are utterly irrelevant to these disorders.

Sixth,

We physicians are brought up with the *double-blind cross-over* paradigm for assessing the results of our therapies. This model is very useful for treatment of acute disease with potent (and toxic) drugs. Symptom suppression with drugs occurs quickly. Drug toxicity usually evolves insidiously.

Nutritional medicine calls for *outcome-based* assessment of clinical results obtained with nutritional strategies. The treatment of disease with nutrient protocols is designed for disease reversal with slow but sustained restoration of physiologic molecular pathways. It does not lend itself to assessment with the double-blind cross-over methods.

I discuss these subjects in detail in the sections on *The Dogma of the Three D s* and *The Dogma of the Three Boxes* in the chapter on *The Cortical Monkey and Healing* in this volume.

Cellular pathology and molecular pathology.

Virchow wrote *Cellular Pathology* in 1858 and liberated us from the constraints of gross pathology of ancient and medieval times. Now *molecular pathology* must liberate us from the constraints of cellular pathology. Cellular pathology shows the cellular damage *after* it has occurred. *Molecular pathology* gives us insight about the molecular and electron-transfer events which occur *before* the molecular, cellular, and tissue damage occurs.

Adaptation is a response to environmental change. Once it occurs, it is maintained until a new environmental change forces a new response. It took the physician community some time to adapt to Vichownian thinking. It is to be expected that a similar time-frame would be required for our intellectual adaptation to *molecular pathology*. This indeed is happening.

*The shift from disease to health
requires a shift from cellular pathology
to molecular dynamics.*

Cellular pathology allows us to learn about the cellular damage caused by diseases and permits us to classify diseases on a morphologic basis. But it does not give us much insight into the molecular dynamics which initiate the molecular and electro-magnetic injury. It is of limited value in understanding the true cause of disease. This is true of almost all degenerative, environmental, autoimmune, non-hereditary metabolic, and neoplastic disorders. A growing number of physicians now recognizes this.

In the context of clinical medicine, the essential point is this: molecular medicine cannot be practiced without breaking through the confines of cellular pathology and without basing our therapeutic choices on a sound knowledge of molecular dynamics.

Molecular specificity, Organismic sensitivity.

In clinical pathology jargon, the terms specificity and sensitivity have defined meanings. Test sensitivity is test positivity in disease; test specificity is test negativity in health. The concept of sensitivity is directed at inclusivity, and that of specificity, at exclusivity. Sensitivity of an element in disease means presence of that element in disease; specificity of that element in disease means absence of that element in health. Our prevailing standards of medical care are based on these concepts of sensitivity and specificity. These two concepts are valid in acute disease but not so in chronic disease. In molecular medicine, we need to see the issues of sensitivity and specificity in a different context.

By molecular specificity, I mean accuracy in the knowledge of the structure and function of specific molecules. Molecules must be assigned only those roles which have been soundly established with scientific methods. There is no room for conjecture in this. This concerns the molecules of physiology of fitness, of pharmacology of nutrients, of chemistry of environmental pollutants, of immunology of allergy, of pathology of autoimmune disorders, and of dynamics of self-regulation (and of despair and hope).

By organismic sensitivity, I mean awareness of all the burdens which threaten the integrity of an organism as a whole. These are burdens on our biology caused by internal and external stresses. These are burdens imposed by altered human ecology, ecology of our external environments and ecology of internal environments. These are disorders of an altered bowel ecology, an altered lung ecology, an altered ecology of the urinary tract, an altered ecology of the genital system, and altered ecologies of other body organ systems. Increased susceptibility to microbial infections and autoimmune disorders, in general, occur as a consequence of the above.

Molecular specificity is the anchor of molecular medicine. Specificity in the knowledge of the structure and function of molecules provides the basis for their use in clinical practice of molecular medicine. Organismic sensitivity provides us the context within which molecular specificity finds its clinical applications.

Organismic (holistic sensitivity) requires that we do not test or treat only *parts* of people. Treating colitis with drugs as a *problem of the bowel*, in essence, implies that the bowel exists dissociated from the rest of the body. This also explains why people with colitis never really heal their colon, even when the X-ray and endoscopic examinations show the absence of colitis. People who ever had colitis know this. Colitis resolves only when the inflamed biology of the whole body carrying the inflamed bowel heals.

A clear view of these two concepts of molecular specificity and organismic sensitivity is essential to a clear understanding of the next major issue in molecular medicine: the issue of the double-blind and outcome-based models of research.

DOUBLE-BLIND CROSS-OVER PARADIGM OF MEDICAL RESEARCH

The prevailing research model in medicine is based on the *double-blind cross-over* model. This model has served us well in cellular pathology and in assessing the potency and toxicity of drugs. Drugs exert their effects by blocking, inhibiting, or impairing molecular events in the body. Thus, drug potency and drug toxicity, by definition, are the flip sides of the same coin. On the surface, this may not seem true, but it is readily apparent if we consider the chemical consequences of long-term drug use. It is one of the principal reasons why PDR (Physicians Desk Reference) does not contain a single listing of a drug without adverse effects.

We, physicians, need to recognize at the outset that the double-blind cross-over mode of investigation is not applicable to the clinical practice of molecular medicine.

Protocol of nutritional medicine cannot be blinded. Here I do not refer to the popular (and publishable) short studies of 6 or 8 weeks duration in which medical students or dietitians are used as guinea pigs and fed some diet deficient in one or the other nutrient. Such studies are of no value in molecular medicine. The same holds true for those in classical medicine. If these studies were of any significance to the classicists, they would have no doubt used nutrients for their therapeutic effects. How else do we explain the total lack of interest in mainstream medicine for therapeutic uses of essential fatty acids, essential amino acids, minerals and vitamins?

Protocols of the medicine of self-regulation cannot be blinded. This is self-evident.

Protocols of environmental medicine cannot be blinded. Efficacy of these protocols depends upon the avoidance of molecules which are injurious to a person. We cannot avoid anything unless we know what it is that we are trying to avoid.

Protocols of medicine of fitness cannot be blinded. How does one jump rope for fitness and not know he is jumping rope?

So it is that the results of the popular short-time double-blind studies do not have any relevance to molecular medicine.

If the double-blind method for clinical investigation is not applicable to molecular medicine, what method of research is suitable for advances in molecular medicine? Outcome studies. An outcome study is a study which determines the efficacy of a given set of treatment measures based on the results obtained with those measures. I have discussed these important issues in my book *Nutritional Medicine: Principles and Practice*. See the chapters on *The Principles of Nutritional Medicine*,

RDA: Rats, Drugs, and Assumptions, and *Aging, Accelerated Aging, and Nutrition.*

> ### *The first responsibility of the physician is to teach the masses not to take drugs.*
>
> Sir William Osler

How does a physician heed Sir Osler's advice ? How does he teach the masses not to take drugs if he chooses to dismiss nutritional medicine as a hoax, environmental medicine as treatment of diseases which do not exist, and self-regulation as a simple-minded and wishful pursuit ?

> ### *When the only tool a man has is a hammer, everything looks like a nail.*

If we physicians turn our backs on the possibilities of nutritional medicine, environmental medicine, and the medicine of self-regulation and healing, all diseases appear to be drug deficiency syndromes, to be treated by supplying the missing drugs.

Moving to Molecular Medicine

I meet physicians who recognize they are treating diseases and not patients, with an alarming frequency and with serious qualms. They are disillusioned with the practice of a medicine which so often *treats* diagnostic labels as it professes to *care* for the patients. These are physicians who recognize the limits of cellular pathology. They recognize that in classical medicine, their role is to helplessly watch the patient suffer and his disease progress before the tests become positive and they have the green light to use drugs, which often give short-term relief of symptoms and create many long-term problems.

I believe this small group of physicians is bringing forth a fundamental change in medicine. *Physicians of tomorrow will see this not as an evolutionary shift, but a revolutionary change.*

"Doing" replaces caring in the Star Wars Medicine

The Star Wars Medicine is a number-driven and procedure-oriented medicine. It legitimizes and fosters the contemporary paradigm of testing and treating only *parts* of patients. It is ill-at-ease with the essential *relatedness* of human biology. It denies suffering which cannot be numerically quantified. It readily negates the completeness of the human condition when it cannot fit suffering into one of its templates. It severely punishes those who want to practice the healing arts outside its domains. It suffocates common sense. Our medical boards do not take kindly to divergence in medical thought. Our insurance companies look upon preventive medicine with disfavor (it may seem hard to believe, but many of my patients had their claims denied because my office stationery carries the words *preventive medicine*).

Why do we physicians carry such deep distrust of the word *holistic*?

Sometime ago, I had lunch in the hospital cafeteria with a surgeon friend. He talked about the surgical management of a patient with a complicated situation and recurrent cancer. He was interrupted by a page for the O.R. He gulped his coffee, picked up his tray, and said,

"I will see you after I do this stomach."

Doing stomachs, bowels, lungs and uteri, this is the language of the Star Wars Medicine. This is also the *language of the mechanical medicine*. This language reflects a profound change in the philosophy of medicine. *Doing* is replacing *caring* in medicine. Why is this model of doing (testing and treating *parts* of patients) becoming so prevalent? Is it because it absolves its practitioners from the greater responsibility of *caring* for the whole patient? Or is it because the strain of coping with the essential relatedness of human biology is much larger than that of dealing with one body organ at a time. One cannot often use glib diagnostic one-liners in the clinical practice of molecular medicine.

Once a peptic ulcer patient,
always a peptic ulcer patient.

Pathologic Basis of Disease, 1984
Robbins, Cotran and Kumar

The incidence of stomach ulcers has been estimated from autopsy studies to range from one in sixteen to one in six in American males, and from one in fifty to one in fourteen in American females (Gut 1:14, 1960).

The Star Wars Medicine does not have much to offer to the victims of this disease. Stomach ulcer disease is a disease of speeded-up life. Tagamet, Pepcid and other drugs offer only temporary relief. Ask a patient who ever suffered from this disease. The stomach ulcer heals only after the body which carries the ulcerated stomach heals.

In the treatment of chronic disease, Star Wars
Medicine is making the patient, the elephant, and the
physician the proverbial blind man.

Similar statistics can be cited for most degenerative, autoimmune, and non-hereditary metabolic disorders to expand this molecular view of health and disease. Asthma and chronic respiratory disorders, chronic inflammatory bowel disease, recurrent urinary tract infections, many disorders of reproductive organs, arthritis, vasculitis, and sinusitis, are all diseases which can be seen differently in light of the precepts of molecular medicine. There is a large body of data in the literature which fully support the need for a shift from a focus on cellular pathology for treatment with drugs to molecular dynamics for disease reversal with treatment protocols of molecular medicine.

Star Wars Medicine does not heal.
No medicine ever does.

Healing is an innate molecular and cellular function. It has something to do with the energy of life. What Star Wars Medicine does, and it does it well, is to buy time for the injured molecules and tissues to heal with the energy of life. In nature, molecules use this energy of life to self-assemble into new cells and tissues. This is the true nature of the healing process.

Human Ecology

and the Basic Concepts of Ecologic Illness

Environmental illness is rapidly becoming *the single most important chronic health disorder* of our time. The authors of the 1989 Report of the U.S. Preventive Services Task Force elected to exclude any reference to this pervasive disorder in their report. Mainstream medicine also seems to have adopted the approach that this problem will go away if we deny it exists.

Environmental illness usually begins as allergy. It evolves through a variable period of increasing sensitivity to environmental chemicals [formaldehyde, benzene, tetrachloroethylene (dry cleaning fluid), car exhaust, and household solvents are the major chemical villains]. With time, many patients develop autoimmune dysfunctions.

According to the generally accepted medical statistics, one out of five Americans now suffers from allergy. In my own experience, the incidence of allergy is much higher. The true figure is close to one in three.

Environmental illness definitely does not call for Star Wars Medicine. Indeed, in my clinical work, I regularly see patients devastated with the tools of such medicine (frequent abuse of antibiotics, steroids, and immunosuppressant drugs).

We live on an alien planet.

From an ecologic standpoint, we live on an alien planet. The air we breathe is polluted. The water we drink is contaminated. The foods we eat are often laced with pesticides, antibiotics, and hormones. Within this century, we have brought upon ourselves chemical and electromagnetic avalanches.

The planet earth has been our habitat for a long time. Homo sapiens, our species, adapted well to the earth environments during this period. Our water remained uncontaminated. Our air changed but little as we learned to use fire (and breathe smoke). Our diet changed when we moved from the paleolithic (stone age) era to the age of harvesting, about 10,000 years ago, when we learned to farm. These changes, as significant as they were on an evolutionary scale, posed no serious adaptive difficulties for man. Over eons, human metabolism evolved in such a fashion that the oxidant stress produced by metabolism was held in balance by the anti-oxidant elements in man's environments. Man's diet was essentially anti-oxidant in nature. Fruits, vegetables, nuts and seeds afforded man ample supplies of vitamins, essential amino acids, essential fatty acids, and essential minerals.

Human biology cannot adapt
to environmental chemicals rapidly.

We have changed the natural order of things in a short period of a few decades. Our science and technology have added chemicals and electro-magnetic burdens which overwhelm our biology. The chemical and radiation avalanches which we have unleashed are devastating in speed and sweeping in range.

The registry of chemicals now lists more than four million chemicals. Over 70,000 of these chemicals are now thought to be in common use in the U.S.A. Most of these chemicals have an enormous capacity to inflict molecular and cellular injury. Only a handful of these chemicals have been studied for this potential. Even when this has been done, it has been done in experimental animals for short periods of time. Our free society thus far has failed to come to grips with this massive problem.

The sad truth is that we, men of medicine, have been most derelict in this area.

The concept of multiple chemical hypersensitivities as
a disease entity in which the patient experiences
numerous symptoms from numerous chemicals and
foods caused by a disturbance of the immune system

lacks a scientific foundation.......As defined and presented by its proponents,multiple chemical hypersensitivities constitutes a belief and not a disease.

A.I.T., Professor of Medicine
Occupational Medicine. Volume 2, Page 693
Philadelphia, Hanley and Belfus, Inc. 1987

Man's Existence on Planet Earth is Fragile.

The possibility of irreversible damage to man's biology (even extinction) by the ecologic changes alluded to above has not gone completely unrecognized. Enlightened biologists, anthropologists, ecologists, and physicians have increasingly recognized the dangerous environments we are creating for ourselves and our future generations.

Yes, I agree chemical hypersensitivity is a belief. I believe I can help patients made sick by exposure to chemicals in their environments.

Francis Waickman, M.D.
Chairman, CME Committee, American
Academy of Environmental Medicine.

The notion that man is predestined to survive is being

challenged. A vast majority of life forms which ever lived on our planet have become extinct. From an evolutionary perspective, it is naive to think that man will not succumb to the same pattern. Could it be that we are unwittingly hastening that process?

THE ENVIRONMENTAL ILLNESS SYNDROME

The prevalence of sick buildings varies by country. Up to 30% of new or remodelled buildings may have high rates of complaints.

Professor Thomas Lindvall
Karolinska Institute
report of WHO subgroup on the
"Sick Building Syndrome", in
Clinical Ecology, 3:140, 1986

The results reveal a consistent doubling of the rate of medication treatment for hyperactive/

inattentive students every four to seven years
such that in 1987, 5.96% of all public elementary
school students (in Baltimore county) were
receiving such treatment.

> Journal of American Medical Association
> 260:2256, 1988

So we drug our children for discipline. What is this new
malady of hyperactivity and inattentiveness? Why is it growing
among our children as an epidemic? We first label
inattentiveness as a disorder. Next, we accept it as a disease
to be treated with drugs.

I have discussed in detail the disorders of the Sick Building
Syndrome, Hyperactivity Syndrome and many other syndrome
caused by environmental exposures in my book *The Dog and
the Dis-ease Syndrome.* Here, in the context of the Star Wars
Medicine, I include a brief sketch of some ecologic concepts of
human disease.

THE ALTERED BOWEL ECOLOGY SYNDROME

I use the term *Altered Bowel Ecology Syndrome (the ABE
Syndrome)* to refer to a complex symptom-complex in which:
- symptoms are attributed to various organ-systems;

- symptoms are attributed to various organ-systems;
- pathogenesis of symptoms can be attributed to molecular events which either occur in the bowel or are profoundly influenced by bowel ecology;
- various morphologic patterns of cellular and tissue injury are seen in the gut as well as in some distant anatomic location; and
- reversal of cellular damage and relief of symptoms cannot be achieved without restoring the bowel ecology to its native state.

In the *Altered Bowel Ecology Syndrome,* I include some well-defined pathologic lesions as well as some entities which are well-characterized clinically but their pathologic basis are not yet well understood. The former category includes morphologic variants of the chronic inflammatory bowel disease, ischemic bowel lesions, and other types of colitis. The latter category includes food and mold allergy, disorders of altered bowel transit time, absorptive dysfunctions, the so-called *Candida-related Complex,* and parasitic infestations of the bowel which, in general, represent secondary events.

BOWEL: THE TRUE INTERFACE

In the preface of this book, I wrote that man has two windows to the world around it: the human brain and the perspective, the immune system is infinitely more important of the two. From an immunologic perspective, the human bowel is the true interface between the human organism and the world around it. It is the bowel lining which separates an internal order from an external disorder. It is this organ which allows the human biology to distinguish between what is *self* and what is *non-self*. We are now beginning to recognize the essential nature of the local gut immune system. The bowel is not just an absorptive surface.

The respiratory tract also serves as a similar interface, but not to the same degree. As environmental pollution increases, indeed it may approach bowel in its importance in the causation of immunologic injury.

The human immune system exists as a plant rooted in the soil of the bowel contents.

What sets *The Altered Bowel Ecology Syndrome* apart from many other disorders is the multiplicity and complexity of pathophysiologic processes involved.

With some exceptions, *The Altered Bowel Ecology Syndrome* evolves over a long period of time during which the patient neglects signals from a bowel in duress, or drugs are used to suppress the symptoms. Resolution of this syndrome and restoration of bowel ecology to a normal state must also be looked at as a slow and sustained process. This is the crux of looked at as a slow and sustained process. This is the crux of the matter. Simplistic attempts *"to get rid of the yeast"* are yet fraught with more dangers.

The treatment of this disorder must be individualized carefully. Recognition and treatment of co-existing allergic and environmental disorders, auto-immune dysfunctions, and metabolic and nutritional deficiency problems are essential to the goal of restoring the bowel ecology to its normal state. The issues of hydration, bowel transit time, metabolic roller-coaster, and stress are all critically important.

THE ALTERED LUNG ECOLOGY SYNDROME

Sheila suffered from a diffuse and generalized skin rash for many years. When she consulted me, I saw serum oozing from large angry raw skin lesions on her thighs, buttocks, low back, arms, and abdomen. She found the simple act of sitting painful. She had suffered from multiple food, mold, and pollen allergies. She knew she was sensitive to chemicals but did not know the identity of chemicals which affected her.

"Sheila, when was the last time you went to a fabric store?", I asked her.
"Oh, I must stay away from fabric stores." she replied.

"Why?" I pursued.

"Because the last time I was there I developed a severe asthma attack and I had to be taken to the emergency room for an adrenaline shot."

This is a dramatic example of the illness triggered by events (formaldehyde exposure in this instance) occurring in the ecology of the lung. I see less dramatic examples of this phenomenon every week.

Formaldehyde is used to enhance the texture of new fabrics. Formaldehyde also is one of the principal chemical villains of our time. According to the Formaldehyde Institute of America, 5 billion pounds of formaldehyde were produced annually in the mid-1980s.

THE ALTERED SKIN ECOLOGY

Omar, our son attends Boston College. Two summers ago, he worked as a laboratory assistant in Jackson Laboratory in Maine. Twice during the summer he visited us. He observed that his general skin condition and acne seemed to deteriorate in direct relationship to the distance from Teaneck, New Jersey. His acne cleared completely during his stay in Maine. His acne lesions reappeared when he was in Boston and it became most intense during his stay in Teaneck.

It is not unusual for ecologically aware physicians to see this phenomenon among their patients from the Caribbean islands. The incidence of skin lesions (acne, dermatitis, rashes, and fungus infections) rises among these people when working in the U.S. and it falls when they return to their islands for extended visits.

Environmental pollutants are major chronic excitants for skin lesions. Should it surprise us? Plants succumb to environmental toxins. Animals sustain injury from exposure to chemicals. Metals and stone exposed to the environments corrode. Why should human tissues, cells, and molecules be impervious to the corrosive powers of pollutants?

THE ALTERED URINARY TRACT ECOLOGY

Helen consulted me for undue fatigue and a general sense of ill being. During her initial visit, I asked her how often she had taken antibiotics in the past five years. She replied,

"I was forever taking antibiotics for
bladder infections, for one month out of every
three, may be for two months out of four, until I finally
figured it out."

"You know, I read a book about bladder
infections written by a woman who suffered from these
infections. I learned to drink lots of cranberry juice and
take lots of vitamin C and some other vitamins."
"And now ?" I asked.
"Now, I don't take antibiotics anymore."

I see an increasing number of patients who relate such case
histories to me.

This basic concept of looking at disease as altered ecology
of a given set of molecules, cells, tissues, organs, or an organ-
system is, in essence, the central theme of my concept of
molecular medicine.

MEDICINE IN BOOTHS

Here is how one of my physician-friend sees the future of
Star War Medicine:

*"Medicine will be all corporate. There will be tall
buildings full of computers. There will be small booths
for physicians. Computers will make all the diagnoses
and decisions. Doctors will write their prescriptions out*

of booths, a booth for the bowel, a booth for the lung, a booth for the uterus and a booth for the head. Human touch and trust, as we see it today, will be no more."

This is not one physician expressing his deepest concern. Such talk is pervasive in our hospitals these days.

People as pets

If the present trends were to continue, my friend's prediction might come true. Indeed, it has occurred to me if the man-machine interface might slowly evolve into relationship in which computers will keep people as their pets. I have wondered about this, but I really don't think that is likely to happen.

I see Star Wars medicine differently.

A DIFFERENT FACE OF STAR WARS MEDICINE

In an illness, what populates our imagination evokes biologic responses. Suffering creates compelling images of yet more pain, more intense suffering, more advanced disease. Can suffering create equally strong images of healing and health?

My patients speaking in this book and the companion volumes, *The Pheasant and Suffering in Illness* and *The Dog and the Disease Syndrome*, give clear answers to this most central of all questions in self-regulation.

In a way, Star Wars Medicine is a moving picture which is only beginning to come into focus. Pain, anger, suffering, passion, cellular and molecular injury, and healing, all are electro-magnetic events. The high-tech of Star Wars Medicine is giving us the means to generate, record, and reproduce these events.

There is a difference.

In this new molecular medicine, information developed with the high tech of Star Wars Medicine is not used as a license for drug therapies. Rather, it is used to direct and precisely target the non-drug treatment protocols of molecular medicine.

Accurate and precise information is essential for the patient if he wishes to know his disease at a *biologic-limbic* level. Knowledge at this deeper level is necessary for disease reversal with protocols of molecular medicine on a long-term basis. It is also necessary if patients are to understand the futility of the hope in classical medicine that chemical (drug) solutions to the dominant chronic problems of our time must be accepted as the *prevailing standards of care.*

I foresee that Star Wars Medicine will continue its conquest of acute disease affecting *parts* of people (legs, sides, or trunk of the elephant touched by the blind men).

I also foresee that Star Wars Medicine will allow us to ever so clearly observe the essential *relatedness* of human biology (the whole elephant).

Patients are being taught self-regulatory methods using advanced computerized electro-magnetic technology, high resolution microscopy of living, breathing, and moving cells, computerized electro-dermal technology, and microphotographs for precise, true-to-life imaging directed to their specific cells and tissues in duress.

Molecular data produced with highly sensitive diagnostic technologies are being used to allow patients to understand their disease at levels that even physicians could not only a mere two decades ago.

The central issue in Star Wars Medicine is not how to use Star War technology; the issue is knowing when not to use it.

Our anesthesia is safe. Our surgery is highly skillful. The issue is not how to operate on people safely. The issue is how far should we support the patient with protocols of molecular medicine so he does not need safe surgery? Tissues after surgery are never quite the same as they were before it.

Our diagnostic technology is highly specific and sensitive for detecting tissue injury. Our synthetic molecules are very potent in arresting the various biologic processes. The issue is not how to effectively deploy these tools of Star Wars Medicine. The issue is how far can we go with natural molecules (with the treatment protocols of molecular medicine) to restore the molecular and cellular integrity without accepting the long-term consequences of chemical interruption of physiologic molecular pathways?

The true promise of Star Wars Medicine.

The Star Wars technology allows us to detect molecular and cellular injury at a very early date. The issue is not how to excel in labelling such injury. The issue is how to understand such early molecular injury, and how to reverse it by restoring, by natural means, the molecular mosaic which is health. This, to me, is the true promise of Star Wars Medicine.

*Nothing must be said or written that
diminishes the likelihood that
someone else will get
at the truth.*

Sir Peter Medawer

Section 4

Lata
and Limbic Breathing

*There is more wisdom in your body
than in your deepest philosophy.*

Nietzsche

Limbic breathing is a specific mode of breathing for self-regulation and healing in *auto-regulation*.

In *limbic breathing*, each breath is taken to achieve some well-defined objectives. In early training, a person uses *limbic breathing* to become aware of the process of breathing. Next, *limbic breathing* is practiced to dissolve the feelings of anxiety and anger, and to control the stress response. With more training, *limbic breathing* is used to learn control over the functions of heart, arteries, brain, skin, and other organs. With still larger experience, this mode of breathing is the most effective method for the initial work for self-healing. Finally, *limbic breathing* ushers a person into higher states of consciousness.

In the working model for self-healing which I call *auto-regulation* in this book, I use the term *limbic state* to refer to a state of the human condition which is necessary for success in self-regulation and healing. Since awareness and practice of the specific mode of breathing in auto-regulation is essential for clinical results, it seems appropriate to call this type of breathing *limbic breathing.*

The emphasis on the role and efficacy of breathing in the various methods for self-regulation is not new. The ancient masters considered breathing as the core activity for self-healing. The central role of various breathing methods in meditative techniques of Egyptian priests, Hindu yogis, Bhuddist teachers, Tibetan lamas, Christian monks, and Muslim sufies and dervishes are well documented.

The language of biology is energy. Language of molecules is oxidation and reduction. Oxygen breaks molecules down to smaller sizes and releases energy for various life processes; reduction builds them back and stores energy. Oxidation, by and large, requires oxygen. We breathe oxygen to sustain life. I have discussed the essentials of the chemistry and energy generation at the cell membrane in the companion volume *The Dog and The Dis-ease Syndrome.*

What is often not fully understood is that the mode of breathing, and the rate of oxygen introduced in our metabolic pathways with it, profoundly influences our state of biology.

The task for me in my work with *auto-regulation* has been how to select, adapt and adopt breathing methods so as to render them easy to learn for my patients. The issues for me have been clinical relevance and efficacy. Further, I clearly saw the need for precise measurements and reproducibility in my work with these breathing methods.

Three Observations about limbic breathing.

For the *limbic mode* to heal, it must first be freed from the relentless censor of the *cortical mode*. Switching off the thinking *cortical mode* is simple to understand at an intellectual level, but it requires considerable practical skills in real life situations. The harder one tries not to think, the more difficult it becomes. This is a universal experience. *Limbic breathing*, when mastered and practiced frequently, is the simplest and most effective method for shutting out the unrelenting chatter of the *cortical mode*.

Three events stand out in my personal observations of *limbic breathing*. Each event brought me an important insight into the place of *limbic breathing* in self-healing. Each event led me to test the validity of this idea with several of my patients suffering from a variety of health disorders.

THE FIRST OBSERVATION

I made my first observation during a period of experimentation with various methods of breathing. I was trying to see how far I could stretch the breathing cycle. I drew a line on a paper each time I breathed in. When I finished this period of test breathing, I felt rested and charged with a high level of energy. I calculated my rate of breathing by dividing the number of lines on the paper by the number of minutes. It turned out to be nine breaths for every five minutes. That started me wondering. What was the state of my body metabolism during this period of breathing?

This observation of a high energy level resulting from a period of very slow breathing is quite intriguing. According to the prevailing and generally accepted concepts of human metabolism, we need oxygen to generate energy. Slower rate of breathing should give us a lesser amount of oxygen. A lesser amount of oxygen should reduce the level of energy.

At the rate of nine breaths taken during a period of five minutes, I took in about one eighth as much oxygen as I would have with my usual pattern of breathing. With this drastic reduction in my oxygen intake, my tissues should have been oxygen-starved. I should have felt weak and energy-depleted. Yet, I had made a personal observation of a very high level of energy resulting from a period of slow breathing. Where did this energy come from? To what was this apparent paradox due? How might I understand and explain this phenomenon? These questions remained with me for several weeks.

At a superficial level, one can assume that a very slow rate of breathing can cause deep relaxation, and so reduce the need for energy for the basic biologic functions. In standard medical terminology, we call this the basal metabolic rate, but there is a deeper question here. It is one thing to conclude that slow breathing lowers the basal metabolic rate. It is another thing to try to explain why an individual should observe a much higher level of energy with this technique. I have discussed the scientific basis for this phenomenon in the companion volume *The Pheasant and Suffering in Illness.*

THE SECOND OBSERVATION

I made the second personal observation about breathing while Talat, my wife, and I were returning home from our office. She was driving. I started experimenting with different modes of breathing. At one point I wondered if I could feel my right hand swell up as I shifted my breathing awareness to it. By this time I had acquired a fairly precise control over my *pulses*, and was able to freely change the patterns of circulation in my hands and other parts of my body. An ability to open up the arteries in hands and other body organs is a very basic and useful skill in auto-regulation. It brings extra blood to the tissues, warms them and gives a clear and pleasant sensation of heaviness. See the section on *The Directed Pulses* in my book *The Pheasant and Suffering in Illness.*

During this experiment, I felt a warming effect and a throbbing sensation in my right hand within a short period. Within several minutes, I felt the effect I had hoped for. I felt my right hand swell up each time I breathed in. Next I tried the same approach with my left hand. Again it worked. I felt my left hand swell up each time I breathed in. Encouraged by this insight, I explored several other parts of my body. I felt my right leg swell up with inhalation. I followed it with my left leg and then thighs, and then stomach and other body organs. Each time this effect was more pronounced than the preceding time. I decided to extend this observation with some of my patients.

This skill of enhanced perception of body tissues, and ability to selectively change the intensity of such perception, came naturally and effortlessly to some of my patients. For other patients with indolent and debilitating illnesses (those who needed *limbic breathing* the most), I was to find out later, it proved to be a very demanding task.

THE THIRD OBSERVATION

I made my third personal observation about *limbic breathing* in the coffee shop of the Ramada Inn in New York City. That evening my wife, Talat, and I saw Baryshnikov play Gregor in Kafka's *The Metamorphosis*. It rained hard as we stepped out of the theatre. We walked two blocks and thought of getting out from under the rain. We went into the coffee shop and asked for some tea. As we waited for the tea, I decided to go limbic, and this is when it happened. Of all places, in a busy mid-town Manhattan coffee shop.

In the coffee shop I was not prepared to make an all out effort to reach the *limbic mode*. I just felt like doing some *limbic breathing*. Each time I breathed out, I did so slowly, evenly, and with full awareness of my limbs, my torso, my face, my head, and other tissues, all at once and simultaneously. It was not my considered decision to reach for an intense awareness of all tissues concurrently. It just happened so. I stayed in this state with the *limbic breathing* for several minutes. The waiter put the tea pot on the table with a loud thud. I opened my eyes. At that moment I realized I had been in the true *limbic mode*.

This was the very first time I had been totally devoid of all thoughts, and, yet, I had been deeply aware of all the tissues in my body throughout this period of time, the life and energy and vibrancy of living tissues. Evidently, the intense awareness of the impact of the *limbic breathing* on my body tissues had completely freed my *limbic mode* from the unrelenting censorship of my *cortical mode*. Quite unintentionally and unwittingly, I had succeeded in achieving the goal which had eluded me for such a long time. There was an important lesson in this:

We can forever think and struggle to shut out the cortical mode, and stumble in the "cortical tunnels". Or, we can use simple methods to bring about a change in the state of our biology which allows us to escape into the limbic openness.

We do not have to be sequestered in Tibetan mountains to

be able to reach the *limbic mode* at will. It is possible to do so in a busy life in a modern city. Serendipity taught me this important lesson. After this initial observation, I put myself to test on several different occasions. Most of the times I succeeded without much difficulty.

THINKING ABOUT HOW NOT TO THINK: A CATCH 22

In our model for self-regulation and healing, the entry into the *Limbic mode* requires that we ablate all *cortical thoughts*. This is easier said than done. This is a classic catch 22 situation: thinking about how not to think. It is a competitive effort. All competitive functions are *cortical* functions; trying hard not to think assures continuity in thinking.

The *limbic mode* arrives when we allow our biology to change. This is what occurred in the Ramada Inn. Even though I had become quite proficient in the various *auto-regulation* methods by this time, I still found it difficult to slide into the *limbic mode*, consistently and predictably. Caught off guard and out of a competitive mode, I went deep into *limbic breathing* and slipped into the *limbic mode*.

CORTICAL BREATHING

A person breathes 12 to 14 times every minute. If we observe a group of family or friends, we will find that the chest wall and shoulder muscles move up each time they breathe in and move down each time they breathe out. By contrast, the abdomen rolls in each time a breath is taken and rolls out as the air is breathed out. We call this *cortical breathing*, as this is the way we breathe when we engage in our usual *cortical activities*.

In *cortical breathing*, the breathe-in period is short, lasting for about two seconds. It is immediately followed by a breathe-out period which lasts for about three seconds. There is no interval between these two parts of the breathing cycle. Inhalation causes the chest wall to rise; exhalation reverses this movement.The chest and shoulder muscles tense up with breathe-in, and ease off with breathe-out.There is an obvious muscular effort with each breath. Until a person learns to become sensitive to his own breathing, he will be totally oblivious of his mode of breathing. When under stress, and unaware of it viscerally, our breathing rate quickens so that the breathe-in period lasts for less than two seconds and the breathe-out period one second or so. This is a mild form of hyperventilation, a totally unnecessary waste of energy.

Cortical breathing is schematically illustrated in the figure below.

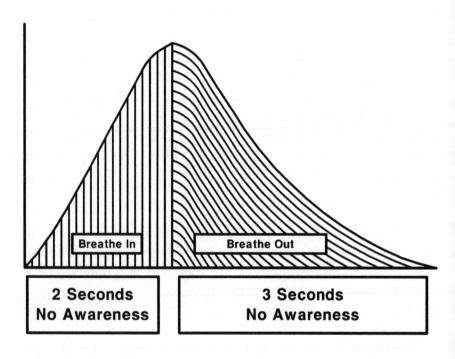

There are three important differences between *limbic* and *Cortical breathing*.

First,

In *cortical breathing*, chest and shoulder muscles contract to pull up the chest wall. The energy expended in doing this work is actually energy spent needlessly. A person breathes about 20,000 times a day. The energy wasted in *cortical breathing* adds up. Unless we understand this and take time to learn to breathe naturally, we are likely to go through our lives wasting a lot of energy.

Second,

In *cortical breathing*, lower parts of both lungs are not as fully expanded and oxygenated as in the *limbic breathing*. This can be confirmed readily by the following simple steps: Put your hands on the side aspects of the lower parts of your chest wall. Next, take a deep breath. Note that the shoulder and chest muscles move up and the hands on the lower chest wall move in. Now take a deep breath while you hold your chest and shoulder muscles still. Note that the abdomen gently rolls out and the lower chest walls moves out in a flare.

Third,

Most importantly, *limbic breathing* puts chest, neck, and shoulder muscles in a restful state. In doing so, it also puts the muscles of the bowel, arteries, and other body organs in a restful state as well. This may not be obvious to someone who has never learned *limbic breathing*, but the truth of this statement will be attested to by all those who have successfully learned effective methods for meditation.

From a physician's anatomic and physiologic perspectives, this truth is also self-evident. As medical students, we are often taught to regard nerves, muscles, ribs, and lungs as discrete organs, but we know that no organ in our body exists alone. No cell is an island by itself. Every cell, every tissue, every organ in the human frame is structurally and functionally integrated with every other cell and tissue and organ.

CORTICAL LIVING GIVES US CORTICAL BREATHING

Cortical living is living in the head. It is chronic thinking. Chronic thinking begets chronic worrying. Subservient to the dictates of the head, the body organs suffer and suffocate. *Cortical living* is head-fixation, and head fixation gives us *cortical breathing*, tight arteries and tight muscles. *Cortical breathing* tires the chest and shoulder muscles and punishes the body organs under taut abdominal muscles. Tight arteries and tight muscles starve our tissues of oxygen, nutrient, and energy.

How did nature intend us to breathe? To know this, all we need to do is to watch a sleeping baby breathe. A sleeping baby breathes naturally and effortlessly. When the baby breathes in, his abdominal wall gently rolls out. As he breathes out, the abdomen gently rolls back. His chest wall moves but little. His body muscles stay limp and loose.

A physician can usually diagnose pneumonia in a sleeping baby by simply observing his breathing mode from across the room. A baby with pneumonia labors for each breath. As he breathes in, his chest and shoulder muscles move up and out; these muscles move down and in when the baby breathes out.

The basic mode of breathing of person under stress is the same as the baby with pneumonia, albeit less pronounced.

UNLEARNING IS SO MUCH HARDER
THAN LEARNING

We have a choice. We can breathe naturally and effortlessly, as a sleeping baby does. Or we can breathe *cortically*, work our chest and shoulder muscles needlessly, keep our abdominal muscles taut, and unknowingly punish our body organs.

Years of *cortical breathing* create breathing patterns which may be hard to break. It requires patience and perseverance to change this. I see this in some of our patients. The concept of not making an effort for a breath is totally alien to them. Breathing like a baby becomes an intellectual pursuit for them. Letting the diaphragm muscles do what these were designed to do becomes a difficult chore. What is so natural for a baby becomes so demanding a task for the grown ups. Unlearning is so much harder than learning.

TRAINING IN LIMBIC BREATHING

To simplify training in *limbic breathing* for my patients , I have divided this mode of breathing into three levels: a beginner's level, an intermediate level, and an advanced level.

To reiterate, the purpose of *limbic breathing* is not to simply become good at its mechanics, though that is essential. The objectives in *limbic breathing* are to feel the full biologic effects of this mode of breathing and, with time, to be able to relieve the burdens on biology which cause the *Dis-ease Syndrome* and disease. This is an important practical consideration. It is necessary for a person to be proficient at the basic methods of auto-regulation before beginning the practice of *limbic breathing*. If he has not learned these methods, he should do so with the help of a tutor.

BEGINNER'S LIMBIC BREATHING

In *limbic breathing*, we learn to allow the chest wall to

move naturally and without restriction. This permits the chest cavity to open up and let the air in, again naturally and without restriction.

"---the lung therefore opening like a pair of bellows draws in the air in order to fill the space."

Leonardo da Vinci

The natural mode of breathing is regulated by the natural movements of diaphragm, the sheet of muscle which separates the chest from the abdomen. The diaphragm *knows* how to move evenly and effortlessly so that the breathing can be even and effortless. The *cortical activity* is an acquired habit, a poor way of breathing imposed upon the body tissues by the *cortical brain*. In *cortical breathing*, the chest and shoulder muscles are needlessly punished with each breath.

Limbic breathing for the beginners is schematically illustrated in the figure below.

Beginner's limbic breathing

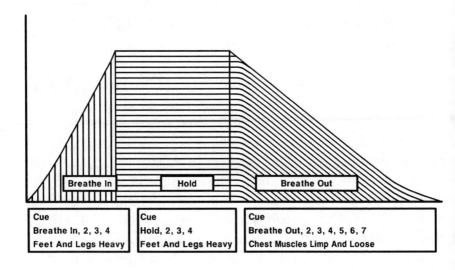

Cue	Cue	Cue
Breathe In, 2, 3, 4	Hold, 2, 3, 4	Breathe Out, 2, 3, 4, 5, 6, 7
Feet And Legs Heavy	Feet And Legs Heavy	Chest Muscles Limp And Loose

In the diagram drawn above, the relationship and the duration of the three phases of a breathing cycle are given in a schematic way. The breathing cycle in this mode of breathing is separated into three distinct phases:

A phase of "Breathe-in"
A phase of "Holding breath"
A phase of "Breathe-out"

In the breathe-in period, a person learns to pace his breathing. He slows his rate of breathing by prolonging both the breathe-in and breathe-out periods. I teach my patients to count three as they breathe in, hold their breath as they count two, and count four or five as they slowly breathe out. After each breath in this fashion, I ask them to take three or four breaths in their usual way. Next they repeat the slow breathe-in and breathe-out periods with counts as described above.

After a few minutes, I ask them to change the method for slow breaths. Now they mentally repeat the phrase " my right hand is heavy and warm " twice as they breathe in. Next they mentally repeat " my right hand is heavy and warm " twice as they hold their breath. Finally, I ask them to breathe out slowly and evenly as they mentally repeat the sentence " my chest and shoulder muscles are limp and loose ".

A person learning *auto-regulation* needs to breathe in this way for a sufficient period of time so that he can achieve the spacing and the duration of the three steps effortlessly. At this stage he also needs to acquire sufficient control over his patterns of circulation so that he can observe the effects of hand warming. If necessary, hand warming can be objectively documented with the use of a suitable inexpensive electronic skin temperature device.

How long should a beginner stay with the beginner's *limbic breathing* before progressing to the Intermediate *limbic breathing*? There is no fixed time for this. From experience I know that this will require little effort for some and persistent attempts by others. This much I can say without reservation: Every body does succeed in this.

There are two objectives in the training for Beginner's *limbic breathing.*

First,

To learn to be sensitive to and become comfortable with the cycle of *limbic breathing.* In this cycle, the breathe-in period is even and short. It is followed by a brief period of holding the breath. Next follows a period of slow, even, and sustained breathing which may last for twice as long as the breathe-in period.

Second,

To learn to warm hands and bring throbbing or the *pulses* to one or both hands during the breathe-in and hold periods. During the breathe-out period, the objective is to feel limpness and looseness in the chest and shoulder muscles.

LABOR OF BREATHING

In some individuals, a slower rate of progress in learning *limbic breathing* is to be expected. These people are used to labored breathing. Natural, effortless breathing becomes foreign to their nature.

People with a high level of tension, anxiety and stress often fall into a pattern of shallow and rapid breathing. This is, in reality, a mild form of hyperventilation, a state of respiratory burn-out. These individuals face immediate, albeit temporary, difficulty when they are asked to breathe at a slower rate.

There is another subset of people who live in a metabolic roller-coaster. The swings between the "highs" and "lows" of this state may be triggered by faulty nutrition, food allergy, chemical sensitivity, altered gut ecology, emotional factors and a host of other causes. The rapid hypoglycemic-hyperglycemic shifts caused by missed meals and sugary snacks are commonly encountered disorders. Lack of sufficient water (dehydration) often compounds these problems. Again, a slow and even mode of breathing represents a change and, hence, a discomfort, for them. I have discussed this subject in considerable detail in my book *The Dog and The Dis-ease Syndrome*.

Smokers usually find such training difficult and laborious. Smoking causes irritation of the bronchial tubes, induces spasms of the bronchial muscles, and increases mucus production in these tubes. Eventually, smoking damages the lung tissue causing ballooning of the air sacs in lungs, commonly referred to as emphysema. These structural changes, however, occur quite late. It seems to me that the principal difficulty experienced by smokers in early training in *limbic breathing* has more to do with the state of their biology rather than any structural changes caused by smoking.

Recent research has shown significant abnormalities in the brain receptor chemistry of smokers with severe cigarette addiction (and also among subjects with drug addiction). It seems likely that the disorders of brain receptors in such individuals which lock them into cigarette and drug addiction also hold them into captivity of the *cortical mode* and *cortical breathing*.

" DR. ALI, NOTHING HAPPENS. "

Caesar, a hospital worker in his late thirties, consulted me for chronic " ileitis " of several months duration. He looked exhausted with pain and stress.

Several months earlier, his physician had diagnosed Giardia lamblia (a type of intestinal parasite) based upon a positive stool test. He was given courses of Flagyl and some other anti-parasitic drugs. After some initial relief, his symptoms of severe abdominal pain and cramps returned with increasing intensity.

Caesar had suffered from asthma for several years for which he had been prescribed a number of different drugs. He knew he was very allergic. His allergies, however, had not been diagnosed or treated.

During the months before he saw me, he had developed increasing tolerance to pain-killers. His symptoms had become disabling and his work very difficult for him. He looked exhausted with pain and stress.

After diagnosing his allergies with micro-Elisa blood allergy tests and some other necessary tests, I put him on our allergy and nutritional protocols. I also gave him training in *auto-regulation*. I gave him copies of my two booklets describing the various theoretical and practical aspects of *auto-regulation*.

I explained to Caesar that his allergies, asthma, and ileitis, were all facets of his basic biologic problem: an immune system put under strain by his genetic make-up, and now laboring under multiple burdens of allergy, asthma, parasitic infestation, drug use, unrelenting stress of pain and disability, and an altered bowel ecology. The diagnosis of " ileitis " was in reality a bowel weighed down by these burdens.

Patients in captivity of painful chronic disorders often are uncertain about the treatment methods of their physicians. This uncertainty, not infrequently, grows into suspiciousness when they are not familiar with the proposed treatment. Caesar was no exception. I recognized he had deep doubts about my approach with allergy and nutritional protocols. The concept of *auto-regulation* appeared to be very unsettling for him. He made no attempts to hide his bewilderment and discomfort at my treatment strategy. Caesar knew of my pathology work at the hospital and that I had personally examined several thousand biopsies of the bowel performed for inflammatory conditions. Except for this, I thought, he would have moved on to yet another physician.

Weeks passed by. Caesar was regular with his nutrient

protocols and allergy injections. He read and re-read the two *auto-reg* booklets. He did *auto-reg* with and without my tape. His condition continued to deteriorate. I offered him the option of drugs commonly used for ileitis. He declined that. I felt compelled to prescribe a strong pain-killer to give him some temporary relief.

The practice of *auto-reg* seemed to be a mechanical chore for Caesar. On one visit he said with evident bitterness, " I do *auto-reg* regularly. But I do not feel any throbbing. I do not feel any *pulses*. I do not feel any energy. It is very frustrating. Dr. Ali, nothing happens."

I sometimes wonder how often patients recognize the many doubts and uncertainties which their physicians live with everyday. I began to wonder if I would ever be able to help Caesar dissolve his ileitis. It was clear to me he had not bought into *auto-reg*. Nor did he show any convictions about my attempts to restore his bowel ecology to its normal order. I reviewed his entire case one day with him, hoping for a break somewhere. He appeared dejected. He complained how he had read the *pulses* book again and done the tape several times. He had completely failed to feel the *pulses* each time he had tried very hard to do so. And then he said,

"I guess I should tell you what happened the other night when I did *auto-reg*. I finished the tape. It did relax me, but I did not feel any pulses or throbbing. After the tape, I did some breathing. I do not know if you would call it limbic breathing. After sometime I felt a sudden intense flush in my arms and hands. Then I felt a sharp sense in my feet. My wife is a registered nurse. I called her and asked her to feel my swollen hands."

Caesar had missed the whole point of *auto-reg*.

The core idea of *auto-regulation* is to listen to one's biology, and be prepared to receive a response from it. *Auto-regulation* is about healing energy. Any tissue response is an expression of this energy. In *auto-regulation,* we build on such a response. When our tissues do respond, we do not ask anyone else to feel it. There is no other elusive goal.

After weeks of fruitless efforts, when caesar's biology did respond, he missed it cold. As I explained the significance of all this to Caesar, I saw more clearly than at any time before the difference between talking for control and listening for healing. The former creates noise and clutter and pain and suffering; the latter brings calmness and relief.

ONE LIMBIC BREATH, THREE REGULAR BREATHS.

Many people find *limbic breathing* difficult during initial training. The feel air hunger as they try to slow down their breathing rate. This is especially true of patients with asthma and other breathing disorders. People with anxiety disorders often get used to a mild form of hyperventilation and experience some difficulty in changing their pattern of breathing. A simple method to overcome this difficulty initially is to take one *limbic breath* and follow it with two or three regular breaths. This sequence can be repeated throughout the period of *auto-regulation.* In most cases this simple trick is enough to break the initial barrier to *limbic breathing.*

LIMBIC BREATHING FOR CHILDREN

Sandra was only 19 months old when she learned to control her asthma with limbic breathing.

Sandra suffered from food allergy soon after she was born. She developed full-blown asthma attacks before she reached her first birthday. She was on regular doses of theophylline (a broncho-dilator drug used for asthma control) and required multiple additional daily doses of another medication with an inhaler to control asthma attacks. Like most other children with asthma, she developed frequent infections and had been treated with antibiotics on several occasions.

After making the diagnosis of food, mold and pollen allergies with micro-elisa blood tests, I put her on our allergy desensitization and nutritional protocols. I also excluded certain food items from her diet. As the frequency and intensity of her asthma attacks diminished, I gradually reduced the dose of her drugs. In 13 weeks, her asthmatic symptoms were completely relieved. At this time, I discontinued all drugs.

I knew that *complete* control of asthma without drugs requires success in all three types of protocols of molecular medicine (allergy, nutrition and self-regulation). Every time I saw Sandra in our office for an allergy injection, I tried to think of a method for teaching Sandra *auto-reg*ulation. Every time I drew a blank. She was obviously too young for me to engage in a discussion of my concepts of *cortical and limbic modes*. It was obvious that I could not explain to her how her air tubes (bronchi) tightened to cause asthma attacks, and how she could loosen them with *auto-reg* to ease her breathing. I had to improvise.

Sandra's mother often brought her two older children to the office. They would play with Sandra as if she was their doll. One day I saw them hold Sandra by her arms and lift her up with swinging movements. That opened up a window for me.

I cannot explain to her how to attend to her bronchi. What if I taught her how to attend to some other part of her body that she can relate to? What if I then taught her how to "transfer" that awareness to her bronchi?

I recognized I could not relate to Sandra at an intellectual level. But then that was not necessary. Obviously her older brother and sister related to her quite well, at a level Sandra understood well.

I called Sandra's mother to my consultation room. I explained to her how I was going to approach the problem of teaching Sandra *auto-reg* for normalizing her breathing if asthma ever recurred. I told her to start playing a *limbic game* with Sandra and her other two children at home. In this game, they will stand in a circle, half stretch their arms, and hold each others hands. Then they will raise their hands gradually and gently breathe in for three seconds (the breathe-in), keep their hands up for two seconds (the hold period), and then very evenly and slowly breathe out for four to six seconds (the breathe-out period). After two or three regular breaths, they will repeat the sequence. I explained to Sandra's mother this would help Sandra to learn pacing for *limbic breathing*. It will also seed the core idea of *auto-reg* in Sandra's mind.

When a person attends to a part of his body, it responds.

A few weeks passed by. Sandra came down with a cold and developed wheezing. That is one her mother and two siblings tried the *limbic game*. Sandra dissolved her asthma attack, for the first time without drugs.

At the time of this writing, Sandra has been free of asthma and drugs for over eighteen months.

Auto-regulation comes easier to children. They do not carry any load of disbelief. They need not unload the burdens which they do not carry in the first place.

A THOUGHT BECOMES A MOLECULE

How they can I change my body functions and heal my disease simply by doing *auto-reg?* Patients often ask me this question during training in auto-regulation.

I have often wondered why we raise this question when we see our thoughts change into molecules every moment. Indeed, life would not have been possible if this was not so.

Let us put this to a simple test. Please, look at the number of the page of this book you are reading, close the book, pause for a few moments, open the book again at the same page, and read on.

I asked you to do a simple test. You agreed. This thought of agreeing with me and following my suggestion produced thousands of molecules in your body. You moved your eyes to see the page number, you moved your arms and hands to close the book, your eyes moved again as you paused, and you moved your arm, hand, and finger muscles to open the book again. All these physical changes could not have taken place without your body producing thousands of molecules, enzymes, neuro-muscular synapse transmitters, and lower energy-bond molecules (to release energy for these muscle movements). Does the same phenomenon hold for brain waves, heart rhythm, and arterial tone? Of course, it does. Our patients, wired with appropriate sensors for electro-physiological equipment observe all this in our *auto-regulation* laboratory every day.

INTERMEDIATE LIMBIC BREATHING

In the intermediate *limbic breathing*, we again have two principal objectives.

First,

To learn to prolong the breath-out period to 10 to 15 seconds, using a step-ladder approach.

Second,

To learn to observe the effects of hand warming and *pulses* in both hands, both feet, all four limbs and the torso, all at once and simultaneously.

The intermediate *limbic breathing*, as the name implies, is a phase between early and advanced training. Many of my patients found it difficult to do the *pulses and feel energy while they learn to* merge the breathe-in with the hold period and the hold period with the breathe-out period. The idea of using a step ladder approach as an interim step came to me while working with a patient.

The Intermediate *limbic breathing* is schematically illustrated in the figure below:

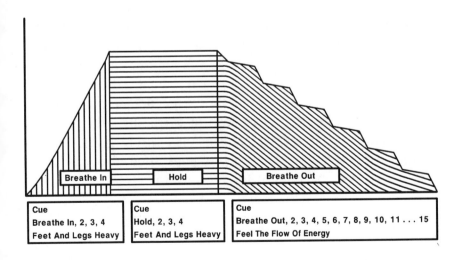

Singing along Lata

The practice of effective breathing methods is central to success with self-regulation. Not uncommonly, my patients find it difficult to learn these methods.

GRACE'S STORY

Grace, a patient with chronic immune dysfunction who had been a smoker for many years, found it difficult to prolong her breathe-out period. She could hold the breath for several seconds, but was not able to make the breathe-out phase slow, even, and sustained. Again and again she tried and failed. I started thinking of a simple method for teaching patients how to prolong the breathe-out phase in a smooth and sustained mode. Thinking, a *cortical activity*, has rarely given me the insights necessary for resolving problems in auto-regulation, so I knew I had to be patient for the answer.

On my way to a medical meeting one day, I was playing Lata Mangeshker on my car tape. I noticed Lata prolonging her breathe-out in that song in an intermittent fashion. That intrigued me. Intermittent breathing, of course, is necessary in most types of singing. Does intermittent breathing have anything to do with the mind-set of the singer? Does the prolonged breathe-out alter the state of biology of the singer? Did Lata's mode of breathing have anything to do with the state of her consciousness? Was that not a good method for a beginner to try? I started singing along Lata. As I had expected, this made my breathe-out intermittent and step-ladder in mode. Next I tried to bring about the limbic effects in synchrony with the song. Again it worked.

After some personal experimentation, I decided to adopt a step-ladder approach to this problem of prolonging the exhalation period. *Intermittent limbic breathing* seemed like a good name for it. So this is how I came to incorporating this simple and effective method for learning the *intermediate limbic breathing*.

It is easier for most people to learn to prolong the breathe-out period as they sing along with a singer. Further, it is easier for people to learn to observe the effects of the circulatory changes concurrently with the effects of *limbic breathing* as their attention is drawn away from the mechanics of breathing. I encourage my patients who enjoy singing along with their favorite singers to learn to be aware of their mode of breathing when doing so. Further, that they add to this an awareness of the *pulses* and perceptions of energy.

Singing along with a song can be considered as an introduction to the method of prolonging the breathe-out period. It has many other obvious advantages. In the context of auto-regulation, however, it should be regarded as a step toward more effective ways of *limbic breathing*.

TAKE A LIMBIC BREATH

Limbic breathing, as mentioned earlier, is the most effective method for turning the *cortical clutter* off. It is also a tricky exercise for the novice in self-healing. It does require practice. One simple method for overcoming this is to do *"minute-reg"*. I have described the concept and practice of *minute-reg* in the section on *The Methods of Auto-regulation* in the companion volume *The Pheasant and Suffering in Illness.*

Go Limbic

Experience with patients suffering from prolonged illnesses has convinced me of the absolute necessity of doing *minute-reg* with *limbic breathing* several times a day. The sicker the patient, the greater the need for it. Of course, it is the very sick who cannot find the initiative and energy to do *minute-reg* frequently during the day. They need frequent reminders. Here is a practical suggestion of proven efficacy. I give one or more of the following signs to such patients with instructions to tape them to the walls of different rooms in their houses.

* *Go Limbic*
  * *Minute-reg*
    * *Take a Limbic Breath*

ADVANCED LIMBIC BREATHING

The Advanced *limbic breathing* is the mode of breathing in the *Limbic State*. Following are the objectives of the Advanced *Limbic breathing*:

An *altered state of the breathing rhythm,* with deep and even breathe-in, a smooth and imperceptible slowing to a complete stop (the hold period), and a very prolonged and sustained breathe-out period.

An *altered state of the brain wave activity,* with a predominance of the alpha-theta rhythm.

An *altered state of the heart function,* with a regular, slow, and even rhythm of the heart.

An *altered state of circulation,* with open arteries, with warmth, heaviness, flushing, a sense of "swelling", and awareness of an intensity of energy in all parts of the body. These effects are most pronounced in hands, feet, limbs, and face.

An *altered state of the muscles* in limbs and torso with dissolution of all tension and strain in these tissues.

In the usual *cortical state*, a person breathes 10-14 times a minute. With *limbic breathing*, by contrast, a person breathes at a much slower rate of 2-4 breaths per minute. He inhales a much smaller quantity of oxygen (20-30 % of the usual amount) than he would with his ordinary mode of breathing.

We should expect that at the slower limbic rate of breathing, we will be oxygen-starved and energy-depleted. In reality, however, the *limbic breathing* restores to our biologic state a much higher level of energy and vigor than is seen in the cortical mode of breathing. This is a simple statement, but the implications of this statement are profound and far-reaching. In its simplest meanings, it shows that *Limbic breathing* alters the state of our metabolism in some fundamental way.

All meditators become familiar with this phenomenon early on during their training in the various modes of breathing. The *limbic breathing* described here, however, is quite different in the profoundness of its effects. In the *limbic mode* of breathing, the profound effects of deep, slow and even breathing are brought in harmony with the total benefits of the changed circulatory patterns and energy perception achieved with the *directed pulses* discussed in the companion volume *The Pheasant and Suffering in Illness*.

The *A*dvanced *limbic breathing* is schematically illustrated in the figure given below:

Advanced limbic breathing

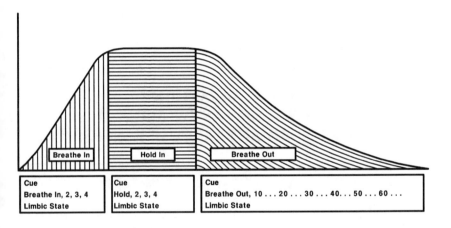

The basic steps in the *advanced limbic breathing* are similar to those in the *intermediate limbic breathing*. There are some essential differences.

In the advanced *limbic breathing* mode, we use all the methods learned in the *directed pulses* to bring forth the full impact of an altered state of circulatory patterns in all tissues of our body. We sustain these effects as we prolong the breathe-out period to 30 to 40 to 50 seconds , or even beyond. This allows long and uninterrupted periods of full awareness of our biologic state with an intensity of perception that effectively precludes all cortical thought activity.

LIMBIC BREATHING: ANY TIME, ANYWHERE, AND UNDER ANY CIRCUMSTANCES.

As with *directed pulses*, practice of effective *limbic breathing* comes easily to some patients, and requires patience and persistence for others. With some exceptions, training in *limbic breathing* is a chore for the beginner. He has to *remember* to breathe with an awareness of the movement of his abdominal wall muscles as well as lack of motion in his shoulder and neck muscles. He also seeks to feel the energy in his tissues as he breathes. He needs to do so 30 - 40 times a day, sometimes even more. With time though, the abdominal muscles adjust to the gentle rolling movement; the chest and shoulder muscles learn to keep still. The resistance melts away. Body tissues respond eagerly.

Seriously ill patients in unremitting suffering, who persist with auto-regulation eventually find the essence of it: Life inside auto-reg is so much more bearable than life outside it.

Many patients with severe, chronic and indolent illness have told me that it is as if they have finally learned to do what they could not do with drugs: make the necessary molecules in just the necessary proportions to relieve their suffering. No chemical overshoot. No rebound phenomenon. No reactive overkill. No adverse effects. This is when *limbic breathing* becomes a way of life. It requires no effort. The individual reaches the goal of *limbic breathing* any time, anywhere, and under any circumstances.

Biologic Profiling with Limbic Breathing

The ancient masters seem to have understood, by pure intuition it appears, human biology and the impact upon it of the various self-regulatory methods. However, only a very few perceptive and intuitive individuals could do so. Even then, it took them decades to perfect these methods. The pupils would spend a life-time of servitude to their masters for such learning. There was one other important difference: these yogis, dervishes, and priests, by and large, lived the lives of hermits. There were no issues of " control over time " for them. Life had not been " speeded up " yet. Nor did they face the problem of what to do with the time they saved by speeding-up their lives.

Most of us live lives which are different from those of ancient masters. Our self-regulatory methods must be different as well. We do not have access to their simple living, but they did not have access to our technology.

I teach my patients *limbic breathing* in my auto-regulation laboratory using a variety of electro-magnetic technology. In these methods, sensors for blood oxygen saturation, lung function, heart, pulse height, skin electro-magnetic conductance, muscle energy, and brain waves are attached to the patient. I have two objectives:

First,

To see objectively the changes which take place under the skin of the patient as he learns *limbic breathing*.

Second,

And equally important, to allow the patient to see these changes, as they appear and disappear, on the computer and video screens, as well as with other suitable techniques. The patient needs to know this, at both intellectual *cortical* and visceral *limbic* levels.

Listening to the tissues for healing. Talking to the intellect for control.

Electro-magnetic and biochemical profiles allow both the patient and the professional to learn how to listen to the tissues and organs for healing. It renders unnecessary, all intellectual analysis about the *role of stress* in the causation of disease. Auto-regulation teaches both the patient and the professional the utter futility of *talking for control* in self-healing. Healing is not a *cortical* function. Healing is a *limbic* phenomenon.

Electro-magnetic and biochemical profiles also clearly establish where the true strength in self-healing resides: with the patient. The physician can only serve as a teacher. No matter how knowledgeable and skillful the physician may be, he can succeed in auto-regulation only through his patient.

Auto-regulation is regulation of self, by self, and for self.

A Cortical Electro-magnetic Profile

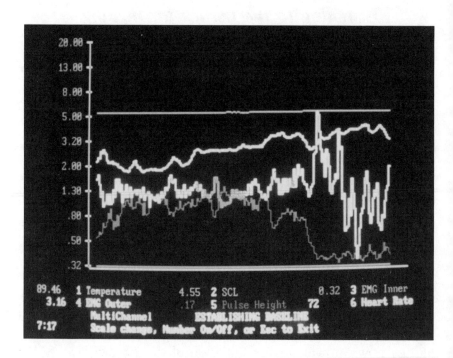

The electro-magnetic profile given above illustrates the changes in biology which I commonly observe in my patients during *auto-regulation* training. The left half of the profile shows a calm, regenerative state while the right half shows a *cortical mode*. It demonstrates body organs under duress. The four lines at the end of the graph indicate from above down: 1) the energy level in the skin (electrodermal conductance response); 2) level of wasted energy in the muscle (measured with an electromyographic sensor); 3) the heart rate; and 4) the state of contraction of the arterial muscle (pulse height measured with a playthysmograph). Note a sharp drop in the arterial line (closest to the baseline) indicating sudden tightness of the arterial wall Tight arteries rob tissues of blood and energy. Tight arteries also make the heart to work much harder as it forces blood through them (shown here by the line just above the pulse line. The toiling heart beats erratically.

A Limbic Electro-magnetic Profile

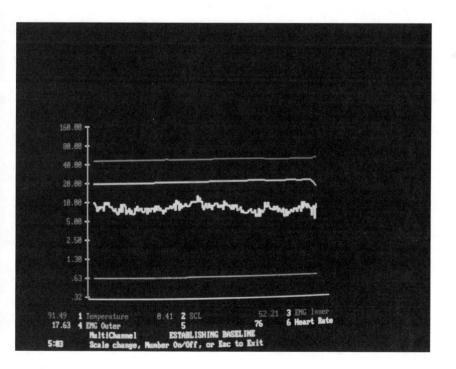

The electro-magnetic profile shown above demonstrates the biology of a patient in the *limbic mode*. The body organs are working at an even pace, in harmony with each other, responsive to each other. The letters in the illustration indicate the same electro-physiologic parameters as in the *cortical* profile illustrated above.

A Biochemical Profile in the Limbic Mode

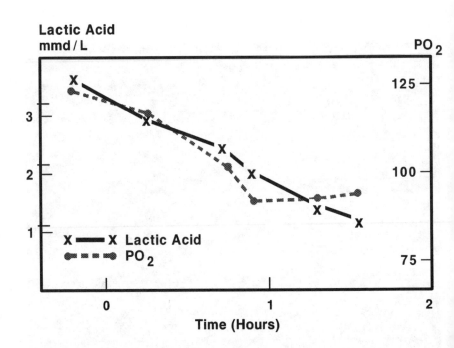

The graph shown above demonstrates the profound biochemical changes one can bring about in his metabolism with *limbic breathing*. The subject in this research study was myself. My collaborator was Madhava Subbarao, M.D., chief of anesthesiology at our hospital. The blood was drawn several times during a period of one and a half hour with an arterial catheter placed in my artery by Dr. Subbarao.

The graph shows a near 75 % drop in the blood level of lactic acid, a near four-fold increase in the blood level of pyruvic acid followed by a precipitate drop, and a sustained drop in the partial pressure of oxygen over a period of two hours. Let us see what these changes mean.

Lactic acid is a molecule produced by cells starved for oxygen. It is an excellent barometer for the tissues under duress.

An olympic athlete knows he has to stop after his peak performance. He knows his tissues will not support any longer the demands of his head. At a biochemical level, his tissue accumulations of lactic acid (and related end-products of metabolism) call a time-out. In technical terms, this is referred to as oxygen debt. With rest, the oxygen-starved tissues are replenished with oxygen and the oxygen debt is paid out. The tissues recover their ability to respond to calls for repeat performance.

An executive shoveling snow in his driveway suffers from a severe spasm of his coronary artery, clogs it with a blood clot and sustains a massive heart attack. His heart fails and is unable to pump sufficient blood to his tissues. As a consequence, his tissues, cells, and molecules starve for oxygen. An oxygen debt develops in them and lactic acid accumulates (commonly referred to as lactic acidosis). The executive suffocates in panic. He gasps for breath. Fortunately he is rushed to the hospital in time. His cardiologist promptly employs potent drugs to dissolve the clot in his arteries. He uses other treatments to stabilize and support the heart, facilitate blood supply to the tissues, and reverse lactic acid accumulation in the tissues. This allows the tissues, cells, and molecules to recover from oxygen starvation. The cardiologist knows that lactic acid accumulation, if not reversed quickly, will further intensify the spasm of the coronary artery and cause death.

A young smoker has a chest X-ray done for persistent cough. He is thought to have lung cancer. His wife panics. The state of panic persists and within hours she develops chest pains. She is sedated and hospitalized for observation.

What could lactic acid and *limbic breathing* have to do with people in these three case histories ?

Drs. Pitts and McLure reported the results of their research linking lactic acid to anxiety attacks and neurosis over twenty years ago (New England Journal of Medicine, 1967, 277: 1329). They administered lactic acid and salt solution intravenously to a group of patients with anxiety neurosis and to a control group. Lactic acid induced an anxiety attack in about half of the patients with neurosis, and interestingly in 20 % of the control subjects. They interrogated these *normal* control subjects and found out that many of them had histories of previous problems. Salt solution used as a control did not cause significant anxiety in either group.

The experience of the olympic athlete gives us insight about how Nature builds its own controls. In health, we must learn to abide by them. Sudden deaths while running seen among ill-prepared joggers are expensive lessons learned when we refuse to heed Nature's signals.

The experience of the executive with a heart attack gives us insight about how cardiologists use the knowledge of lactic acid and starved tissues to treat life-threatening illnesses.

We can learn to reduce our blood lactic acid with limbic breathing. This is, in my judgement, the most precious first-aid kit that everyone can carry with him at all times. One cannot misplace it. It is always there when you need it.

The experience of the wife suffering panic attacks, the research of Drs. Pitts and McLure , and the results of my own research with *limbic breathing* (shown above in the graph) give us insights about the role of lactic acid in our day-to-day activities. Panic and anxiety attacks are two faces of the stress response, the *fight or flight* response of Hans Selye. The stress response is an integral part of our biology, and so is the phenomenon of lactic acid accumulation. We cannot live without these responses anymore than we can live without a brain generating pulses in our skulls.

However, there are things we can do for stress, panic attacks, and anxiety states. We can learn to lower our blood lactic acid levels with *limbic breathing* and other methods of auto-regulation. Indeed, this strategy is the best strategy when our coronary arteries tighten into spasms and we wait for an ambulance. Even a modest loosening of the coronaries with *limbic breathing* in such a setting can give us a survival advantage.

A Blood Gases Profile in Limbic Mode

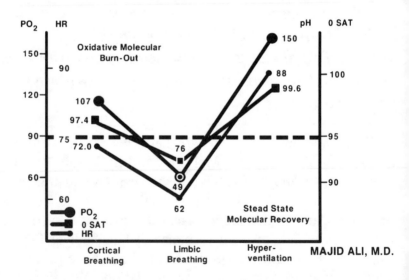

The above graph illustrates the changes in the blood gases seen during three contiguous periods: a period of " normal " *cortical breathing*; a period of *limbic breathing*; and a period of very rapid rate of breathing for deliberately producing a state of hyperventilation.

In the graph above, the line labelled PO2 indicates the pressure of oxygen in the arterial blood. The line labelled O sat indicates quantity of oxygen (saturation of blood) in the arterial blood. The lightly shaded area in the middle third of the graph outlines the region where the molecules are broken down by oxygen to generate energy in health. The darkly shaded area in the upper third of the graph outlines the region of excessive, uncontrolled, and wasteful breakdown of molecules by oxygen in *The Dis-ease State*. I call this the state of " oxidative molecular burn-out ". The un-shaded area in the lower third of the graph outlines the region of diminished molecular breakdown and increased synthesis of molecules in health. I call this a phase of "steady state molecular recovery".

The " normal " *cortical breathing* in this research experiment puts the level of gases in my blood in the "normal" range. Hyperventilation puts the level of gases in my blood in the region of *oxidative molecular burn-out*. In the middle of this experiment, I did *limbic breathing*. The graph shows that the levels of my blood gases were in the region of *steady state molecular recovery*.

The "normal" cortical breathing, in my judgement, is normal only in the sense that most people breathe this way. It is not the optimal way of breathing. By analogy, blood cholesterol levels of 250 - 275 mg/dl were considered "normal" until recently. This was not because that was the optimal level for freedom from premature heart disease, but because most people had cholesterol levels in that range. Now we know better. We want to keep the cholesterol level somewhat below 200 mg/dl and, if possible, substantially below that level.

The graph displayed below shows the data obtained with a second research study. Again, I was the subject under study in this experiment. This graph shows additional parameters of blood pH and blood carbon dioxide levels.

A Blood Gases Profile in Limbic Mode

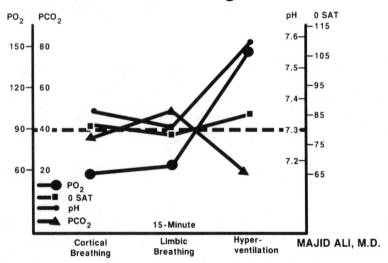

The values for partial pressure of oxygen (PO2), oxygen saturation levels, and pH   fall with *limbic breathing;* the pressure and concentration of carbon dioxide rise to compensate for the changes in oxygen values. These changes reflect a lower rate of metabolism. Oxygen levels fall because the tissue requirements for oxygen decrease. A slow and steady state of diminished metabolic activity allows the body a period for molecular and cellular renewal. This is, indeed, a slowing of the whole process of aging. See the section on *The Agony and the Death of a Cell*   in the companion volume *The Pheasant and Suffering in Illness.*

An Immune Cell Profile in Limbic Mode

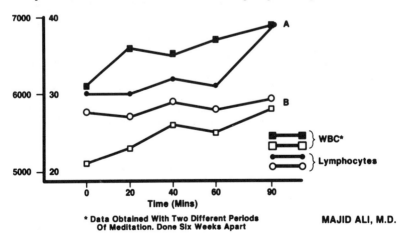

Effects Of Auto-Regulation On Peripheral Blood WBC And Lymphocyte Count

* Data Obtained With Two Different Periods Of Meditation. Done Six Weeks Apart

MAJID ALI, M.D.

The graph given above shows the effects of *limbic breathing* on the number of lymphocytes (the immune cells) and white blood cells (defenders against infections) in the blood. Two lines for each type of the blood cell represent blood cell counts performed during two separate periods of *limbic breathing* on two different days (indicated by letters A & B).

Note that the number of both types of cells in circulating blood rose significantly during both periods of *limbic breathing*. The white blood cell count rose from an initial value of 6100 to 6850 in one test and from 5125 to 5910 in the second experiment. The number of immune cells rose from 32.5 % to 39 % in one experiment and from 21.5 % to 28.5 % in the second.

The changes in the blood cell count appear to be one of the ways by which meditation and self-healing enhances immunity against infections. Parenthetically, I might add that the increases in the blood cell count shown above are very similar to those one expects after a period of exercise.

MINUTE-REG WITH LIMBIC BREATHING

Minute-reg is auto-reg done for a minute or two at a time. I have described the principle and practice of minute-reg in the section on *The Methods of Auto-regulation* in the companion volume *The Pheasant and Suffering in Illness*. Success with *minute-reg* is central to success in treatment of chronic disease with *auto-regulation*.

Minute-reg with *limbic breathing* means just that: breathing *limbically* for a minute or two (or even for less) frequently during the day. Initially, the individual does not perceive any benefits from a few *limbic breath* taken here and there during the day. There are two reason s for this:

First,

> In early training, most people are trying to learn the mechanics of *limbic breathing*. It is simply not possible to feel any *limbic effects* with a competitive, *cortical* activity.

Second,

> In early training, most people are unable to completely ablate the *cortical thoughts* and enter the *limbic mode*.

With training, first with and then without the limbic breathing tape, people succeed in bringing about the profound effects of limbic breathing done for 10 to 15 minutes. It is at this time that the enormous value of *minute-reg* with *limbic breathing* becomes known to the person practicing *auto-regulation*.

This brings me to a point of considerable clinical

importance: the relationship between the *limbic breathing* during regular periods of *auto-regulation* and *limbic breathing* during *minute-reg*. Success in each depends upon the other. Extended *limbic breathing* during regular *auto-regulation* brings us to deeper levels of the *limbic mode* and a greater awareness of the benefits of such breathing. A greater awareness of such effects brings more immediate benefits with *minute-reg*.

I teach my patients not to concern themselves with the presence or absence of perceptible effects within *minute-reg*. *Minute-reg*, even when done for a mere 30 seconds *does* reduce the burden of molecules which put our biology under duress, the catecholamine thermostat. I explain to my chronically ill patients how the common activities of a usual day continuously generate adrenaline and related molecules including the excessive number of free radicals which injure molecules, cells, and tissues. I refereed to them collectively as "oxidative molecules". These oxidative molecules overwhelm the restorative "Life Span Molecules", and cause "molecular burn-out" in tissues. This is the beginning of molecular and tissue injury.

Minute-reg with a few *limbic breaths* prevents excessive generation o such molecules and facilitates their rapid breakdown. The beginner usually is not aware of these changes in his chemistry. These molecular dynamics, nonetheless, do take place. An experienced self-regulator is acutely aware of such beneficial molecular events.

LIMBIC BREATHING FOR ASTHMA

Patients with asthma require a threefold approach for control of asthma without drugs:

1. Protocols of environmental medicine (treatment of mold, food and pollen allergy with immunotherapy (allergy injections), and avoidance of other triggers.

2. Nutritional therapy with protocols specifically designed to stabilize cell membranes and prevent spasm of the bronchial tree and related complications.

3. *Auto-regulation* and *limbic breathing*.

In my experience, optimal immunologic therapy for allergy and appropriate nutritional protocols can be expected to give 60 - 75 % control of asthma without drugs. For complete control without drugs, the patient must learn methods of *directed pulses* and *limbic breathing* and practice *auto-regulation* with regularity.

We recently reported the results of an outcome study of forty patients with asthma at the Advanced Course of the American Academy of Otolaryngic Allergy held in January,

1990 in Phoenix, Arizona. The criteria for inclusion of patients in this *outcome* study were as follows:

1. Patients must have been treated with drugs for asthma for at least one year before consulting us for non-pharmacologic treatment.

2. Patients must have a minimum follow-up period of one year after starting allergy, nutrition and self-regulation protocols.

3. Patients must be enrolled in the study in a consecutive fashion to avoid any selection bias.

The results showed that 29 of 40 patients (72.5 %) who completed the study were completely free of both asthma and the asthma drugs they had previously used. Another 5 patients (12.5 %) used the asthma drugs at an average of less than four times a month. Three additional patients (7.5 %) required drugs 1-3 times a week. Only three patients (7.5 %) were still using the drugs with some regularity. Of these, one patient suffers from cat-induced asthma, has nine cats who often sleep with her, and has made a deeply personal decision not to live without cats. The second patient is an advanced state of emphysema. The third patient had been on steroids for several years with severely impaired immune system before she consulted us.

In this study, we did not make any attempts to establish a double-blind cross-over model for investigation. It was designed to be an *outcome* study.

Auto-regulation cannot be blinded.

In my judgement, the principal weakness of the double-blind cross-over model for research is this: it reduces the patient to a mechanical device, a robot. By blinding the patient, it systematically excludes any role which the patient might, with his own healing power, play in his recovery from his disease. By blinding the physician, it precludes any role which the *patient-physician relationship* may contribute to the patient's recovery. I discuss this subject in the sections on *The Scientific Basis of Auto-regulation* and *The Placebo-busters, Placebo-phobes, and Placebo-philes* in the companion volume *The Pheasant and Suffering in Illness.*

LIMBIC BREATHING FOR HYPERTENSION AND OTHER NON-RESPIRATORY DISORDERS.

High blood pressure (hypertension) is caused by tight arteries. Tight arteries force the heart to work harder. As the blood is pushed through tight arteries, the pressure within these arteries rises. This is the essential nature of hypertension.

The few exceptions to this are some rare tumors and other disorders. Left untreated, hypertension leads to structural disorders of the heart, kidney, brain, and other body organs. In my work with *auto-regulation,* I have found *Directed pulses* and *Limbic breathing* as the two most effective methods for loosening our arteries and normalizing raised blood pressure. Many researchers have shown the efficacy of some other self-regulatory methods for control of hypertension.

Hypertension serves as a good model for many other disorders which can be effectively reversed with self-regulatory methods used in conjunction with treatment protocols of nutritional and environmental medicines.

I wrote in the preface of this book that a surgeon's scalpel seldom heals. An internist's drug seldom heals. Molecules, cells, tissues, and organs have an innate ability to heal. What the surgical knife and drugs do is to remove the impediments in the way of healing. *Limbic breathing* and other methods of *auto-regulation* promote healing in exactly the same way.

I teach *limbic breathing* as an essential part of training in *auto-regulation* to every patient who consults me, regardless of the nature of her disease, intensity of her suffering, or the probability of quick or delayed recovery. This include patients with advanced cancer in whom surgery, chemotherapy and radiotherapy have failed to control the disease or have inflicted additional suffering upon the patient (such patients need *limbic breathing* more than any thing else I know).

LIMCOR

The term " limcor " is my abbreviation for *limbic-cortical balance*. I use this term to refer to a state in which a person learns to do his *day's cortical work with a limbic awareness of his body tissues and organs.*

Modern living is *cortical living*. By and large the burdens of modern life are the burdens of *cortical living*. Some people know this intuitively. They live outside the *cortical barriers* without ever trying hard for it. Others need to learn it. The *cortical mode* loves to analyze, argue, doubt and suspect. It does not let up easily. Indeed, the grip of the *cortical mode* on the body tissues is tightest for those who need the *limbic mode* most: patients in the throes of chronic unremitting illness.

Two issues must be seen clearly.

First,

We cannot go back to living in caves.

Second,

We cannot go on suppressing with drugs the symptoms of chronic disease caused by stress, poor nutrition, food allergy, sensitivity to environmental pollutants, and damaged internal ecology of bowel, lung and other organs. The price paid by the patients for this is prohibitive. So, what then, is the solution?

The concept of *limcor* is neither difficult to understand at an intellectual level nor very hard to use in daily living. *Auto-regulation* is knowledge of biology and an enhanced perception of energy put to work for self-regulation and healing. Nutritional and environmental protocols are more effective when combined with a self-regulatory methods.

Limbic Breathing learned well and practiced regularly is, in my experience, the single best way to achieve *Limcor*.

LIMBIC BREATHING IN TISSUE SENSING

Directed pulses, Limbic breathing, and Tissue Sensing are the three principal methods used in *auto-regulation*. These methods are listed in order of both their complexity and efficacy. In my experience, it is difficult for anyone to practice effective *limbic breathing* until he becomes well-versed with the principles and practice of *directed pulses*. The same holds for *limbic breathing and tissue sensing*.

In *tissue sensing*, one learns to breathe *limbically* and *into* the tissues under stress of injury or disease. It is an advanced and a specific method for self-healing for disorders of specific tissues. It is in the method of *tissue sensing* that *limbic breathing* finds its full value. See the chapter on *Methods of Auto-regulation* in the companion volume *The Pheasant and Suffering in Illness*.

Breathe into your pain and suffering and let go.

Breathing into pain and suffering and letting go? This may appear to be too abstract an idea to be of much practical use in clinical medicine for those who have never explored any methods for self-regulation. In practice it is rather a simple approach. Pain is localized easily by most people; suffering for most people seem to be largely located in chest.

With a *limbic* mode of breathing, we teach patients how to breathe slowly into their chests or in the areas of pain, sensing the energy with each breath (perceived as *tissue rising with energy with warmth, flushing, throbbing, tingling, or pulsing*). *This is followed by a brief period of a few moments of holding breath, still aware of the sense of energy. Next, comes a period of slow, sustained, and even breathe-out period in which that person feels the tissues in the specific area settle down with energy.* This is followed by similar cycles of breathe-in periods with *tissues swelling with energy*, and breathe-out periods with tissue settling down with energy. All during this time, the individual *stays* with the energy in his tissues, and away from all intellectual thoughts.

> *You have to keep breathing into your suffering. If you stop, the suffering returns.*

Richard M., a patient with severe depression.

LIMBIC BREATHING FOR THE SEVERELY ILL

The required frequency for *minute-reg* is determined by the chronicity and intensity of suffering. Some of my patients with severe life-threatening depression have leaned to do this throughout the day. One such patient explained to me how she does this at all time. When asked why, she replied,

> *"Because life outside auto-reg is unbearable"*

I reiterate here for emphasis an essential principle of molecular medicine which I have stated several times in this volume and in two other companion volumes *The Pheasant and Suffering in Illness,* and *The Dog and the Dis-ease Syndrome.* The core idea of molecular medicine is to address *all the molecular events* which threaten the health of an individual. *It mandates that we never test or treat a part of any of our patients.* The treatment protocols of nutritional and environmental medicine must be used in conjunctions with self-regulatory methods for all patients, and for all disorders.

Success with *auto-regulation* for severely ill patients requires patient, persistent, and painstaking efforts. Sometimes, the clinical benefits are maddeningly slow to appear. During this time, it would be very wrong for a patient not to seek all the relief which protocols of nutritional and environmental medicine can offer.

Further, the severely ill patient often needs support with drugs during the initial periods of treatment with *auto-regulation*, nutritional medicine and environmental medicine. This calls for a careful and cautious clinical approach and a close follow-up.

No knowledge can be more satisfactory to a man than that of his own frame, its parts, their functions, and actions.

Thomas Jefferson

Exercises For Limbic Breathing

I have discussed the choice of time, location, body posture, and the duration of auto-reg exercises in the section on *Methods of Auto-regulation* in the companion volume *The Pheasant and Suffering in Illness*. These aspects of the practice of auto-reg are important. It is necessary for the reader to be familiar with these details.

In auto-regulation, words are not important; the effects produced by them are. Words are used only to learn how to attend to different parts of the body so these parts respond to us.

The tone of voice, the emphasis on certain words, the spacing between successive sentences, and intervals between the various steps of this auto-reg exercise are essential for results. I recommend that the reader start with a suitable tape prepared by a professional before making his own tape. Again, the core idea of auto-reg is to learn how to attend to one or more parts of our body. The body does respond. We need not worry about this.

breathing which I use for my own patients. This tape is available from the Institute of Preventive Medicine, Bloomfield, New Jersey. Telephone # (201)-743-1151.

The practice of *Limbic Breathing* and other methods of *auto-regulation,* when used for treating established disease, must be supervised by a physician experienced in principles and practice of self-regulation. I reiterate this here for emphasis. *Safety must be our primary concern.* See the following section on *First, do no harm.*

What is the "on" switch
for auto-regulation

A Kind Feeling

* A kind feeling for body tissues.

* A kind feeling for family

* A kind feeling for friends

* A kind feeling for an animal

* A kind feeling for a flower

* A kind feeling for a field

*In auto-regulation,
feelings heal; reasons do not.*

What is the "off"
switch for auto-regulation.

An Unkind Thought.

Section 5

First, do no harm

*No shrine is holier than the human frame,
for it houses the human spirit.*

Caring for this shrine is a sacred trust, sacred for the patient and sacred for the physician. It is this trust which sets medicine apart from other professions.

Physical disrobing of a patient for examination by his physician is symbolic of a deeper personal and emotional disrobing for the patient. And so it is that the simple act of a physician touching his patient establishes a unique bond between the two. This bond must not be breached by any expediency.

Molecular medicine is not an easy way out for the poorly informed physician. It is not an excuse for an exemption from the labor of learning and knowing. Knowledge of the molecules of physiology of fitness, of pharmacology of nutrients, of chemistry of environments, of immunology of allergy, of pathology of autoimmunity and of biology of self-healing - these are the essentials for the practitioner who takes this less-travelled road of molecular medicine.

Molecular medicine is not an easy way out for the patient either. It calls for an abiding trust in his physician. It asks for an ongoing pursuit of the knowledge of a patient's own biology. It requires a diligent search for all the stressors on his biology. It shifts the focus away from a chemical resolution of the burdens on biology. It draws the patient toward natural methods for molecular recovery and renewal. It requires recognition of all the physical and chemical triggers of his illness. It requires a different mind-set, a change from a talking mode for control to a listening mode for healing.

First, do no harm

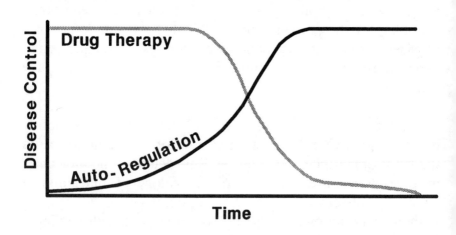

This is the first principle of classical medicine. This is also the first principle of molecular medicine. Indeed, it must be regarded as the first principle of all disciplines in medicine. In molecular medicine, this principle puts substantial additional responsibility on its practitioners. Practice of molecular medicine requires a much deeper understanding of the human biology than is necessary if our goals are simple relief of symptoms with drugs.

Success with protocols of molecular medicine comes naturally and effortlessly to some patients, and it requires diligent and persistent efforts by others. The core issue is this: no disease must be allowed to progress while a patient learns the principles and practice of molecular medicine.

For patients receiving drug therapy, the dose of the drug must be titrated cautiously with progress made with nutritional protocols and other therapies in molecular medicine. Drugs must be discontinued safely, and only after the patient has had substantial experience in control of his disease with self-regulation protocols.

Diseases afflict people differently. Diseases damage tissues differently. Diseases evoke healing responses differently.

Diseases hurt people differently. People hurt by diseases express their hurts differently. Different hurts require different remedies.

The goals in molecular medicine must be defined clearly. The goal may be reduction in the dose of a drug used for a specific disorder. It may be discontinuance of the drug. It may be control of symptoms which cannot be controlled without drugs. It may be a decision to postpone surgery. Finally, it may be a considered decision to avoid surgery altogether. Whatever the goals, these must be understood and agreed upon by both the patient and the professional.

In my own clinical work, I adhere to some fundamental principles of molecular medicine which I described in my book *Nutritional Medicine: Principles and Practice.* I reiterate here two essential principles.

First,

Never test and treat only a *part* of a patient. In Molecular Medicine, one does not just test and treat a bit of the bowel for colitis, a slice of the stomach for an ulcer, a shred of the synovium for arthritis or a clip of the coronary artery for the problems of the heart. This would be in a fundamental conflict with the precepts of molecular medicine.

Second,

Never withhold from the patient any of the supportive treatment protocols of nutritional and environmental medicine, and the methods for self-regulation, and fitness. These protocols must be used concurrently and with equal emphasis.

In this book and in the companion volumes *The Pheasant and Suffering in Illness* and *The Dog and the Dis-ease Syndrome*, I have related several case histories. Some of the results I describe appear to strain credibility. For the first few years of my work in molecular medicine, I went through long periods of uncertainty and self-doubt. The results I observed with protocols of molecular medicine (without using drugs) were far superior to those obtained with drugs and described in medical texts. A large number of my patients who had been maintained on multiple drugs (including steroids) for several years were able to stop these drugs completely *and* obtain complete relief of symptoms. The case histories included in these volumes are true to life. Only the names and gender of the patients have been changed.

During the last few years, many of the physicians who attended my workshops for molecular medicine, and who tried some of my protocols, have obtained similar results. This peer review has been very valuable to me. It has sustained me during many periods of conflict between the concepts of classical medicine and the precepts of molecular medicine. It is an important point, and I have reiterated it several times in this book. As more physicians incorporate protocols of molecular medicine in their clinical practices, I know they will make similar clinical observations.

There are several other clinically significant issues. There is the issue of the role of molecular medicine in acute disease and in chronic disorders. There is the issue of important differences between the way drugs exert their effects and the way molecular protocols work. There is the issue of anticipated time-frames of efficacy of pharmaceuticals and molecular protocols. I address these issues at length in my book *Nutritional Medicine: Principles and Practice.*

*Disease reversal with molecular medicine is
fundamentally different from treatment
of disease with drugs.*

The patterns of relief of suffering with molecular protocols
are fundamentally different from those observed with treatment
of disease with drugs. Molecular protocols include treatment
protocols of nutritional medicine, environmental medicine,
medicine of self-regulation, and medicine of fitness.

Drugs, I indicated earlier, act by blocking, inhibiting or
impairing the various enzymatic pathways and electromagnetic
events in human biology. Drugs are designed to do so with
speed and efficacy. Thus, symptom suppression with drugs is
expected to occur within a short period of time. This also
explains why *all* drugs will sooner or later exhibit adverse
effects. The Physician's Desk Reference does not contain any
listing of a drug which does not cause symptoms of toxicity.

Restorative treatment protocols of molecular medicine, by
contrast, work by replenishing the various molecular pathways
of human metabolism. This is, in general, is a relatively slow

process. Where drugs begin to exert their effects within hours, nutritional, environmental and self-regulatory protocols begin to show their effects in days, sometimes in weeks. This is an element of considerable clinical significance. The patient must be prepared for this.

There are two other important aspects of disease reversal with molecular protocols (and without drugs): an aspect of initial and limited worsening of symptoms, and an aspect of the essential fluctuating nature of the recovery process. I illustrate them in a schematic fashion below.

The Disease Reversal

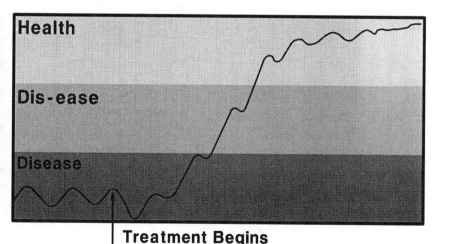

In the above diagram, the curve for disease shows a drop (indicating an increase in the symptoms and suffering) as treatment begins with molecular protocols. I observe this phenomenon with high frequency in patients with chronic indolent disorders. Fortunately it lasts for a short time, rarely lasting for more than a few days. It is not always clear to me why this happens. The likely causes are initial and limited gastrointestinal nutrient intolerance and changes in bowel ecology.

The second more important aspect of this model of disease reversal is the essential fluctuating nature of the healing process, the "highs" of symptom relief and disease remission are followed by "lows" of symptom recurrence. Some of these highs and lows are biologic in nature, and are integral to the essential nature of the healing process. Other highs and lows occur because the patient begins to take liberties with the treatment protocols; the symptoms gain in severity as he omits treatment protocols, and subside as he returns to them. However, each low is followed by a high which rises above the preceding peak. Such highs and lows notwithstanding, the patient makes sustained progress.

To cure sometimes, to relieve often, to comfort always.

Anonymous

Section 6

The Cortical Monkey
and
Healing

Putting something
between the monkey and his wound.

There is a species of monkey in Karnal, my birthplace. During my childhood, these monkeys lived in our town by the hundreds. They were a nuisance for the grown ups, but for us children, they were a lot of fun. I remember my father telling me how these monkeys had a peculiar habit. They did not let their wounds heal.If one of them ever lacerated his skin, he picked on his wound continuously. Whatever little scab did form, he would peel it off. These wounds festered for long periods of time.

It has occurred to me that the first man to invent a bandage probably got his idea from watching a monkey (or some other animal) constantly pick on his wound. It might have occurred to him that the way to let the wound heal is to put something between the monkey and his wound. When he got hurt himself, the lesson learned from the monkey might have taken a practical turn. A bunch of leaves, perhaps of some herbal plant, might have served this purpose. This , or something closely similar, is likely to have been the beginning of the idea of the primitive bandage, the forerunner of our band-aid.

In my working model for self-regulation and healing in clinical practice, I use the term *cortical* to refer to an aspect of the human condition which calculates, competes, cautions, creates stress, causes immune dysfunction, and culminates in disease. I use the term *limbic* to refer to a state of the human condition which cares and comforts, creates images of health, and heals. I have discussed this subject at length in the chapter on *Beyond Positive Thinking: Two States of Human Biology* in my book *The Pheasant and Suffering in Illness.*

There is something of relevance in the story of Karnal monkeys to our ideas of self-regulation and healing. Time and again, I see patients who understand how their *cortical condition* throws road-blocks in the way of *limbic healing*. I demonstrate to them their biologic profiles composed of a host of electro-magnetic or molecular events in our *auto-regulation* laboratory. I show them how their whole biology is sustained in an even state when they go *limbic*, and how it is thrown in turbulence when they go *cortical*. I explain to them the impact on their internal organs of *talking for control* and *listening for healing*. At intellectual and analytical levels, they observe all these and seem to understand them. Yet left to their own designs, they slide back into the calculating and competitive *cortical state*. They are unable to keep their analytical mind (the *cortical monkey*) out of their healing *limbic state* .

Indeed, at times it requires patient and persistent work to break long-established *cortical habits* and put the *cortical monkey* to sleep.

Thinking is an intellectual function;
healing is not.

In auto-regulation, I do not ask my patients to think positively. In *auto-regulation*, I strive to teach them *how not to think*. Thinking about how not to think is a classical catch 22. The harder we try not to think, the deeper we slide into thinking. This is where the concept of energy in *auto-regulation* comes into play.

The theoretical concepts of the value of positive thinking are well understood by most people. The obvious benefits of positive thinking notwithstanding, such thoughts by themselves, in my experience, are rarely sufficient to allow most people to reverse chronic disorders and regain health. Indeed, for patients debilitated by chronic diseases and exhausted by chronic suffering, the advice of positive thinking is often a cruel play on words. I do not do this.

Auto-regulation is healing with energy;
it is not healing with counselling,
analysis, regression, hypnosis
or biofeedback.

The concept of physical healing energy in *auto-regulation* is often misunderstood in a society oriented to chemical resolution of all health problems. Many of my patients relate it to some variant of Eastern philosophy or mysticism when I introduce them to the principles and practice of *auto-regulation.* Fortunately, most people are able to perceive this healing energy in some fashion or other during the very first training session in my *auto-regulation* laboratory. This strips the concept of healing energy of most of the layers of disbelief, distrust, and apprehension. From then on, it is simply a matter of increasing the intensity of such energy and enhancing its clinical benefits.

Injured molecules and cells heal with energy. Auto-regulation is about this energy.

The critical issue here is how to become aware of this energy, how to increase its intensity and, finally, how to use it to regulate one's biology and allow the injured molecules and cells to heal. In the initial stages, it is necessary to understand clearly what *auto-regulation* is and what it is not.

Auto-regulation is healing by listening to tissues and perceiving their energy.

Auto-regulation is not healing by talking to tissues and thinking positively.

The principles of self-regulation are valid for all patients and all diseases. The applications of these principles, however, require careful evaluation of each individual patient to assess the nature and extent of his disease (weight and duration of the specific burdens on his biology).

Different diseases cause different levels of suffering, and require different degrees of effort with different timeframes.

We Americans are a numerical people.

We love numbers. We cherish them. We live by them. We are sustained by them. When deprived of them, we crave them. We seek safety in numbers. Without our numerical crutches, we are vulnerable.

Modern medicine is a numbers game. Numbers tell us how to label our pain. Numbers define the magnitude of our suffering. Numbers give us our diagnostic labels. Numbers give us our treatment strategies. We conduct research with numbers. To generate our research numbers, we happily blind ourselves. Dissatisfied with simple blinding, we invent methods to *double-blind* ourselves.

The numbers generated by our medical diagnostic laboratories should serve us as sign-posts; instead, we joyously submit ourselves to their servitude. In medical school class-rooms, we insist that our students become physicians who *care* for people and not treat their laboratory test results; in clinical wards, we *treat* diseases with numbers. We dare not defy the numbers. When challenged, we rise to defend our numbers. When no other defense holds up, we invoke *defensive medicine,* a medicine where the prey is not the patient but the physician; the predator is not a disease but a lawyer.

There is a new fever in the country, the *cholesterol fever.* The virus of this fever travels along the radio waves, just as the shingles virus travels along nerve fibers. It is replacing weather as the socially acceptable subject for conversation with total strangers. Some of us, it seems, want to live by our cholesterol numbers. For many, it is an obsession; they insist on their *cholesterol numbers* every few months; some want it every month.

There is much debate about the real threat posed by high cholesterol levels. It seems likely that the cholesterol levels seen in general population will eventually prove not to be a major issue in the causation of heart disease. So many of us are constricting our coronary arteries worrying about our cholesterol numbers. We do this with regularity. How important is the cholesterol level relative to other risk factors for heart disease? What is the ideal cholestrol number? What are the benefits to the heart of lowering the cholesterol level by a few points? What is the potential of harm to the heart which arises from obsessive worrying about the cholesterol level? What is the true cost/benefit ratio here? These essential questions remain unanswered.

We have little understanding of the true significance of the numerical absolutes in the cholesterol story. Yet we happily surrender to them.

We are advised to avoid natural products which contain cholesterol. We are prescribed cholesterol-free margarines and oils which are de-vitalized, de-vitaminized, de-mineralized, de-gummed. deodorized, and bleached forms of fats and oils. Mass-producing technologies take out of these natural products co-factors which are essential for their metabolism and add to them trans-fatty acids (which our body cannot metabolize) and other toxic substances such as aldehydes, epoxides, and cyclic compounds. These trans-fatty acids and other toxins sit on our cell membranes just as a candy-wrapper sits on a mountain trail for years because the soil does not know what to do with plastics. There is one important difference: the soil may eventually recover from the ecologic disruption of plastic materials in some centuries; our cells do not live that long.

To lower the cholesterol number, an ever increasing number of us are taking drugs and eating foods packaged as *cholesterol-free*. Drugs lower cholesterol levels by disrupting lipid metabolism. What are the long-term consequences of such chemical intervention? We will not know this for several years.

Now for cholesterol-free foods. The issue should be what is good nutrition and not how to achieve or maintain a certain cholesterol number. If cholesterol in natural foods really was so toxic to man, Eskimos would have become extinct a long time ago. Our forefathers would have suffered a similar fate.

Isn't it odd that the incidence of heart disease and other degenerative disorders seems to be rising in parallel to the use of so-called cholesterol-free foods in our diet?

Good nutrition is a matter of mind; it is neither denial of dieting nor euphoria of eating. A change in mind must precede a change in food. Dieting does not work because the mouth is not a substitute for the mind.

Some day perhaps we will learn to balance our numerical (*cortical*) prowess for understanding what is outside of our skins with a nomadic (*limbic*) openness for knowing what is under our skins. Then we will be able to look at the cholesterol number without constricting our arteries.

Systemic Resistance

Why do some people effortlessly slide into *auto-regulation* while others struggle and stumble and stop ? No question has preoccupied my mind during my work with *auto-regulation* more than this question. I have spent endless hours working with my patients searching for an answer to this. Evidently, a key to this puzzle would be very valuable in advancing self-regulation as a valid medical discipline.

In my work, I can count on my fingers the number of patients who seemed to have much intellectual difficulty with the principles and practice of *auto-regulation*. I give formal instruction to my patients in the methods of *auto-regulation* for self-regulation and healing in seminars specifically designed for this purpose. It is evident from their questions that they fully understand the subject matter and its implication in preserving health and treating disease.

So I will dismiss at the outset a failure of comprehension of what auto-regulation is and how it works as the major cause of common initial difficulties and very rare eventual failures.

There are two real issues here.

Cancelling the cortical clutter.

And

Learning to listen limbically.

Auto-regulation, I indicated earlier, is self-regulation and healing with *energy,* the energy of molecules and tissues. It is not healing with the commonly held *mind-over-body* view of coping with disease.

Not uncommonly, I observe in my patients an initial visceral resistance to perception of tissue energy; long-term difficulties with intensification and use of such energy for healing has been uncommon in my work. *It seems to me that when an individual neglects his tissues for a life-time, the tissues sometimes take their time to warm up to him.*

We have speeded-up life (it is not clear to me what we have achieved with the time so saved). *Auto-regulation* initially works by down-grading the accelerated molecular burn-out which characterizes speeded-up life. Here is another catch 22: molecular burn-out which *auto-regulation* is intended to down-grade blocks the way to progress in *auto-regulation.*

Jack Y., one of my patients with disabling environmental illness and the Chronic Fatigue Syndrome, put this dilemma succinctly into common vernacular:

> *"Auto-reg is like credit;*
> *banks will not give it to you when you*
> *need it most. They will throw it at you*
> *when you don't need it."*

Jack Y.

Indeed, it is hard to quieten the mind when the body hurts. Tissues in pain acquire a louder voice as we begin to listen to them. This is how the suffering, not uncommonly, intensifies as a patient begins *auto-regulation*. Some of my chronically ill patients wanted to give up *auto-regulation* for this reason. With continued practice, however, tissues in pain do respond and suffering abates.

> *Serious illness changes you for the better,*
> *if it does not kill you first.*

Robert A.

Most patients with seriously chronic illnesses learn to listen to their tissues in duress. A few patients are fortunate enough to do so with guidance from professionals. Most others learn to do this by trial and error. Rarely, patients do this intuitively. No one wants serious illness so he can change for the better. But when we do fall victim to a chronic indolent illness, the option of self-regulation carries this promise.

The Cortical monkey: A great masquerader

The *cortical monkey* has many faces and wears many masks. There is a mask of disbelief, a mask of fear, a mask of anger, and a mask of defiance. Then there are masks of *false hopes, guilt of failure,* and the *placebo effect.*

A faucet in stomach

Juan is a Spanish construction worker in his early fifties. I first saw him when he brought his son to see me for allergies and undue lassitude. During the visit I realized he (father) needed care more urgently than his son. His gastroenterologist was treating him for a large stomach ulcer diagnosed with endoscopy. His urologist was treating him with repeated courses of antibiotics for prostatitis. An otolaryngologist had diagnosed chronic sinusitis and prescribed yet more antibiotics. He suffered from intractable lower abdominal cramps and low back ache for which he was prescribed yet more drugs.

Like many fathers, Juan seemed to intuitively know that his son was following his footsteps in his vulnerability to illness. Like most parents, he seemed anxious to avert that at the expense of ignoring his own health. I chose not to discuss my impressions of his health problems with him. When his son gets better, I thought, he would want to get treated too. His son had multiple allergies, and appeared to be under considerable stress. With our protocols for nutrition, allergy, and *auto-regulation,* he was much improved within a few weeks. Now the father was ready to start.

Diagnostic work-up for Juan was simple and straight-forward. The treatment of his problems turned out to be anything but simple. Juan could not tolerate my nutritional protocols. Spanish people often suffer from indolent abdominal ailments. He tolerated allergy injections poorly. He did not speak English. I do not speak Spanish. *Auto-regulation* can be difficult when two languages collide with each other. So it turned out to be this time. It was an unsatisfactory session, both for him and me.

For *auto-reg* with imaging, I prepared for him a disease-specific card showing side by side two true-to-life pictures of the inside lining of the stomach wall, one with a stomach ulcer and one without it. He sat, concerned and confused, looking at the pictures. During training in the laboratory, it was the same thing. He looked at his *biologic profiles* which showed moving graphs of his various body organs on a computer screen. He seemed to be trying hard to understand, but with a visible sense of inadequacy .

Turning off the faucet

Weeks went by and he made no progress. One day I drew

a picture of a stomach ulcer. To illustrate the effect of excess acidity in his stomach, I drew a faucet above the stomach ulcer and showed him how this acid was eating through his stomach lining to make the ulcer deeper. I tried to explain to him how he could try to turn this faucet off. He nodded, more in courtesy than in understanding, I thought.

Some more weeks passed. There was no improvement. When a patient does not improve after reasonable efforts, it is only human for his physician to *want* to avoid him. This was beginning to be hard on me. At an intellectual level, I accepted him as my failure. At a visceral level, it was a different matter. I could not stop wondering why *auto-reg* did not work for him.

Some more months went by. I knew his allergy symptoms had improved as expected. I stopped asking him about progress in *auto-reg*.

Self-regulation has its own rewards. Not uncommonly, it surprises us, utterly and totally. One day, out of the blue, he blurted in broken English, " Dr. Ali, I think I can turn the faucet off now."

My progress notes written in his chart 21 months after the first visit include the following quotes, " Feel much better now. No medicine now for stomach ulcer. No antibiotics for prostate trouble. Little back pain. No pain-killers. Vitamin C still bothers. Other vitamin pills O.K."

Why did Juan's tissues refuse to respond for several months? In the end when they did, why did they? What did he mean when he told me he could turn the faucet off? How did he know the faucet was really turned off? These and other questions about Joan's response stayed with me.

THE MASK OF DISBELIEF

The *cortical monkey* commonly enters the stage as simple disbelief.   The premise of self-regulation looks simple and simplistic. The thought that our biology does respond to us and that we can regulate it is foreign to most of us.Indeed, until recently, all such notions were seen as delusional plausibility.

Scientific Skepticism

There are three principal reasons for this: scientific skepticism, absence of knowledge, and prevailing beliefs.

Scientific skepticism among the professionals, in my experience, is the single most important hurdle in the path of self-regulation as a legitimate discipline in medicine. Patients often have read about it and are usually interested in pursuing it. Most professionals have no visceral feelings for it. This is because they have never tried it. Their lack of interest, and sometimes disbelief, becomes evident to the patient even when they do not oppose it vehemently.

The resistance to self-regulation among the physician community is not difficult to understand. Physicians are scientists. Science is measurements and reproducibility. Until recently, we did not have technology for measuring and reproducing the effects of self-regulation on human biology. What could not be measured and reproduced could not be accepted as scientific. Unverifiable claims of success with self-regulation were dismissed as simple-minded or deceitful.

Advances in electro-physiological technology are changing all this. In my *auto-regulation* laboratory, I routinely document the profound changes in various biologic parameters which my patients can affect with *auto-regulation* methods.

Absence of knowledge

Absence of knowledge about the efficacy of self-regulatory methods for treatment of disease is the second major hurdle in this area. Patients often are aware of what has been reported by the media. However, they often regard it as research projects conducted in a university setting, and do not see the relevance of this work to their illnesses. This has not been a very difficult obstacle to overcome in my own clinical work. I give *auto-regulation* seminars for my patients. I prepare tapes and write booklets for this purpose. Most patients learn the principles and practice of *auto-regulation* quickly.

Prevailing beliefs

The third problem of prevailing beliefs poses a more demanding challenge. Prevailing beliefs are usually based on past prejudices, past limitations, and past failures. Such beliefs often are intellectual foreclosures. In times of change in medicine, minority opinion has been right more often than wrong.

Inderal, a crutch?

Joan, a 63 year old woman, consulted me for hives. Her physician had tried to treat her skin disorder with steroids with limited success. She gained weight rapidly with cortisone and was anxious to stop its use. She was also taking Inderal and Isosorbide for attacks of chest pain caused by angina and leg cramps. Her blood pressure was 180/100. With the diagnosis of allergy confirmed with micro-Elisa assay, I initiated immunotherapy and prescribed appropriate nutritional protocols for her allergic and cardiovascular disorders. After three weeks, she developed an intensely painful skin rash of Herpez zoster (Shingles). I taught her *auto-regulation* to control the pain of shingles. She learned *auto-regulation* well and was soon able to dissolve most of her pain with it. In three months, we were able to discontinue steroids. She lost over ten pounds in weight. Next, we started to taper the dose of drugs she was taking for her heart and circulation.

On a follow-up visit eleven months later, she looked very healthy and relaxed. She told me she had not experienced any episodes of chest pain for several months. Her blood pressure was 140/80. There had been no relapse of allergy symptoms. She and her husband were travelling frequently. She was still taking small doses of Inderal and Isosorbide. I spoke about how we could go about discontinuing the drugs altogether. She looked surprised,

"But I have coronary artery disease!"
"You just told me you have not had chest pain for several months," I replied.
"Are you saying the hardening of arteries in my heart is gone?" she looked more surprised.
"No, but it is not causing any problem," I answered.
"But wouldn't it return if I stop Inderal?",
"Do you think Inderal is preventing it now?" I responded.
She kept silent for a few moments.
"Come to think of it, Inderal was not preventing it then," she spoke at length,"it can't be preventing it now."

How many people can discontinue drugs they take for their health problems? How many people continue their drugs needlessly only because of the prevailing beliefs? Later in this chapter I relate the experience of Norman Cousins with his heart disease as he describes it in *The Healing Heart.*

The circle of disbelief about the larger issue of the efficacy of self-regulation in chronic disease grows larger as it feeds off the smaller circles of scientific skepticism, absence of knowledge, and prevailing beliefs.

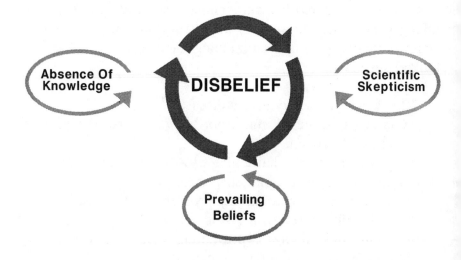

*Self-regulation cannot be prescribed with
a prescription pad.*

Self-regulation must be taught to the patient with patience and persistence. A physician cannot write a prescription for self-healing and a pharmacist cannot dispense it. A physician cannot teach his patient how to slow his heart rate, or dissipate wasteful tension in his muscles, or change his brain wave patterns, if the physician has never done these simple things himself.

It would not have been so bad if the professional would only express his own inability to support his patient in this effort. Not infrequently, he actively campaigns against it, sometimes actually scaring the patient with *his* view of how the disease will progress without drug treatment. He supports his belief with his statistics, all derived with the double-blind cross-over model of research which, by definition, excludes any role that a patient can play in his own recovery. The physician, his statistics, his libraries packed with books, his massive hospitals, his hi-tech tools of the trade, all are stacked against the plausibility of self-healing. The patient, in pain and suffering, usually does not have enough reserves to withstand such an onslaught. He simply accepts drugs.

Clever arteries caution us.

In 1988, Joint National Committee estimated that high blood pressure (hypertension) may occur in as many as 58 million Americans (Arch. Int. Med. 1988;148:1023-38.) It is the foremost risk factor for coronary artery disease, heart failure, stroke, kidney disease, and loss of vision from retinopathy.

What is hypertension? Pressure of blood within the arteries rises when blood has to flow through tight arteries. How do arteries get tight? Arteries tighten when the muscles in their walls tighten. Why do the muscles in the arterial wall tighten? Because they are protesting something. It seems to me that our arteries are very clever. More clever than our brains. They sense and respond to burdens on our biology. They caution us. The only way they know how to caution us is by doing what they were designed to do: constrict. Even when hypertension is caused by rare forms of tumors and immune disorders, it is due to tight arteries. Tumors obviously need to be resected.

What should we do when our blood pressure rises? Listen to our arteries and respond to the burdens on our biology against which they are protesting. What do we do in reality? We numb them with drugs.

A guest lecturer spoke about treatment of hypertension in our hospital. He spent almost the full hour talking about the use of drugs for hypertension with emphasis on his favorite drug. In the end, someone asked him about the value of biofeedback for normalizing high blood pressure. He replied, with evident condescension, that it solves the problem when the problem really does not exist. Translation: when a patient thinks he can lower his raised blood pressure, he is delusional. *We do worship drugs, don't we?* (His favorite drug was manufactured by the company which paid him for his lecture. Pure serendipity?)

Untried Methods
(Untried for those who have not tried them.)

Then there is the warning that self-regulation is an *untried* method. We physicians often go to great lengths to warn our patients against disease progression if they decline the drugs we prescribe. Do we do so because we really know that self-regulation does not work? Or is it because it is easier for us to work off our prescription pads?

There is fairly extensive literature attesting to the efficacy of various self-regulatory methods for normalizing high blood pressure. No one has ever reported any adverse effects of such treatment. Yet, only a handful of patients are ever offered a non-drug, self-regulatory approach with the full support of a physician.

The drugs used for hypertension belong to five major groups: diuretics, beta blockers, calcium channel blockers, ACE inhibitors and centrally acting drugs. As the names of these drugs imply, these drugs act by blocking or inhibiting one or more essential biologic processes. Evidently, our biology was not designed to provide us with beta receptors and calcium channels so we can block them, or the ACE enzyme so we can inhibit it. The ACE enzyme, I might add, is an important enzyme found in a type of immune cells called macrophages. The centrally acting drugs act upon (and disrupt) our center, the brain. Not unexpectedly, all of these drugs have side effects.

To reduce the possibility of premature heart disease in hypertensive patients, we use diuretics, fully realizing that these drugs raise the blood levels of lipids which increase the risk of heart disease.

To solve this problem of hypertension,
all we need to do is to add thiazides
to our water supply.

A professor of medicine, circa 1950

If we do add thiazides to our water supply,
I do not know about hypertension, but every
one will have high triglycerides.

A professor of medicine, circa 1989

Fear feeds upon disbelief, disbelief upon ignorance.

The professionals who deride the role of self-regulation in controlling high blood pressure, in my experience, are always those who never learned it themselves. They oppose something they do not know.

Suspension of Disbelief

Disbelief in the efficacy of self-regulation is rooted deep in the intellectual recesses of our medical thought. We physicians are taught to maintain healthy disrespect for claims of disease reversal with all methods other than the tools of our trade: drugs and surgical scalpels. Some of us actually regard it as heretical.

Suspending disbelief is difficult for every one. Physicians are no exception. To understand this, we need to understand two aspects of the prevailing medical thinking: the "dogma of three D s", and the "dogma of three boxes."

The dogma of three D s
One disease, one diagnosis, and one drug.

In the prevailing medical dogma, we physicians are Oslerian in our thinking: when treating a patient, we search for one disease, strive to make one diagnosis to explain all symptoms, and use one drug to effect a cure. On the surface, it seems a rational, logical, and safe approach. As teachers, we teach this dogma well; as students, we learn it well.

One Disease

One Diagnosis

One Drug of Choice

This dogma of three D s is unquestionably the single most important hurdle in the way of acceptance of self-regulation as a legitimate discipline in medicine, both for the physician and the patient. Indoctrinated in this model of medical thinking, the physician is brought up to search for one disease, make one diagnosis, and prescribe one drug of choice. The patient has been cast in the same mind-set. *He expects one diagnosis of one disease, and wants one drug of choice* to cure him. He is programmed for this, and is troubled if it is not forthcoming.

The first premise of one disease (the first box) leads us to the second premise of one diagnosis (the second box). Little do we recognize that what seems a simple and necessary search for one disease commits us to the not-so-simple notion of one diagnosis. The second premise of one diagnosis inexorably leads us to the third premise of one drug (the third box). Again, the selection of one agent for treatment (the drug of choice) appears to be the next logical, rational and necessary step. This dogma of three D s (a trio of boxes for the mind) seems so right. It is easy to understand how this came to be so deeply entrenched in the prevailing medical thinking.

The dogma of three D s: a legacy of a bygone era.

The dogma of three D s is a legacy of a time when the dominant clinical problems were infectious diseases. It was necessary to look for and recognize a single infective agent and employ the single most effective pharmacologic agent to eradicate it. It was quite common for these infections to present themselves wearing many different masks. By and large, the etiologic organisms responded best to one or two specific drugs. Thus, it was critical to precisely identify the causative organism so that the most effective drug could be used to eradicate the incriminated microbe. In the classical medical teaching, we physicians were trained to be sleuths, and taught to put all the diagnostic data together in such a fashion that one diagnosis of one disease emerges as the only logical conclusion. This paradigm served us well when our enemies were microbes. Tuberculosis, typhoid fever, leprosy, syphilis, malaria, and a host of other parasitic infestations fitted well into this model of medical thought.

Times have changed. The patterns of our diseases have changed. Sanitation and vaccination have been our triumphs over the pathogenic microbes. Infectious diseases are not the dominant chronic disorders of our time in the U.S. and many other countries.

The dominant chronic disorders are not caused by single species of microbes. Rather, these are problems initiated, perpetuated, or compounded by elements in our internal and external environments, elements of bad nutrition, food and mold allergy, chemical sensitivity and toxing, biological consequences of speeded-up life, increased susceptibility to viruses, and immune dysfunction caused by any or all of the above.

*If our chronic disorders are not caused by
individual elements, it stands to reason
that our therapy must not be limited
to correction of just one element.*

✱✱✱✱✱✱✱✱✱✱✱✱✱✱✱✱

To treat is to intervene.

Then there is an even more daunting obstacle in the path of self-regulation. We physicians are interventionist in our upbringing. For us, to treat is to intervene with drugs or with a surgical scalpel. Teaching patients to self-heal is not what we are taught in medical schools.

Young man, go stamp out disease.

So went a popular advice.

It is easy to see why we physicians and patients have so much difficulty with self-regulation, a treatment approach which requires listening and responding, rather than speaking and controlling.

There are yet other obstacles in the path of self-regulation and healing.

Debra's Story

Debra writes poetry and plays for children. She is in her late-thirties. She consulted me for an " immune dysfunction " for which she had been prescribed steroids several months earlier. Predictably, steroids caused weight gain and skin problems. The drug did not mitigate her suffering. She suffered from severe fatigue, muscle and joint pains, and depression.

Debra gave me a long history of a myriad of symptoms of food allergy, mold allergy, and a " collagen disorder. " A collagen disorder, I might add, is a euphemism, a diagnostic label for autoimmune injury. The immune system normally functions to protect an individual against infections, cancer, and various degenerative disorders. To do this, it first distinguishes between its own molecules and molecules which are foreign to it. When stressed, the immune system confuses molecules of its own tissues for alien molecules and produces antibodies against its own molecules. These antibodies, called auto-antibodies, damage its own molecules and cause disease.

I explained to Debra the nature of the various burdens on her biology, and how we could try to systematically identify these burdens and remove them. Specifically, I described to her how *auto-regulation* can be expected to reverse many of these elements at a molecular level. Debra showed intense interest in our protocols of Nutritional Medicine, Environmental Medicine, and *auto-regulation*. Initially she made good progress with *auto-regulation*. She became eager to stop the use of steroids. Then came a period of relapse of her symptoms. She became quite anxious to find the exact name of her "immune disease", and grew increasingly doubtful about the validity of self-regulation.

A few weeks later she called to say that she had consulted another physician who had *finally* diagnosed what her real problem was: fibromyositis. I did not see Debra again.

> *"So many patients came to see us with the diagnosis of fibromyositis that we decided to legitimize it. We know fibromyositis means inflammation of fibrous tissue and muscles which these patients do not have. But then what do you do?"*
>
> A professor of rheumatology lecturing in our hospital.

The dogma of three D s does not give us any insight into the true etiology of any of the common autoimmune disorders. It does seem to give us the comfort of an acceptable model of a disease for treatment with steroids and other drugs. What would happen, I wonder, when patients find out that this is intellectual dishonesty, simple and plain and indefensible?

The Dogma of Three Boxes

The dogma of three D s leads us to the dogma of three boxes: a box of diagnosis, a box of prognosis, and a box of "boxosis". The physician leads the patient into these boxes, one after the other, in general unwittingly. Patients walk into them, one after the other, in general unknowingly. Some patients do fight back, intuitively it seems to me. They rarely succeed. The rush of medical thinking, the promptness in prescription of drugs, the severity in warnings against disease progression if the drugs are declined (the dogma of three D s), are all elements too strong to resist for a person weakened with pain and suffering. Before he knows it he is "boxed-in" tightly within these boxes.

THE FIRST BOX OF DIAGNOSIS

The need for accuracy in diagnosis is absolute. There is no room for error in this. Mistakes made here cannot be corrected later with changes in treatment. This is one of the basic tenets of the classical medicine. *This is also where the major problems in our work as physicians begin.* This is the beginning of the *process of "boxing"*.

Diagnosis

Diseases are burdens on biology. The term *diagnosis* should mean identification of *all* the burdens on a patient's biology. If one diagnostic term could identify *all* these burdens, it would be sufficient. But it rarely does that.

Let us take the case of a man with a fracture of thigh bone sustained in an automobile injury. The term "fracture of femur" as a diagnosis would certainly seem to be an accurate and an adequate diagnosis. Ask any experienced orthopedic surgeon. Healing of the two broken ends of the femur bone after the fracture is set is much more a function of the healing ability of the patient than it is of the surgical skills of the operating physician. The healing ability of the patient is a reflection of the sum total of burdens on his biology: his view of his illness, and perception of his healing process, his nutritional status, his emotional stability, his state of stress, his immune strength, and his resistance to infections.

Now let us consider the case of a young woman with rheumatoid arthritis, a painful, debilitating, and at times, crippling type of arthritis. A physician examines the patient and orders several blood tests and X-rays. The X-ray study shows swollen synovium (the joint lining) and some bone destruction. The blood test for rheumatoid factor turns out to be positive. A diagnosis of rheumatoid arthritis is now *established*. What does the term rheumatoid arthritis really mean here? What does a positive rheumatoid factor test mean? *How is it going to affect the tissues in the joints? How is it going to affect the patient as a person?*

What a patient with so-called rheumatoid arthritis should know is that it is not a disease. It is merely a label. She should know that a positive X-ray only indicates damage to tissues, and not how this damage was caused. What she should also know is that the rheumatoid factor is nothing more than a collection of antibodies. It does not tell her physicians what molecules these antibodies are directed against. In essence, the diagnosis of rheumatoid arthritis tells her nothing but hides much from her.

Once the patient's suffering has been captured in the box of diagnosis, we begin a short trip to the next box of prognosis.

THE SECOND BOX OF PROGNOSIS

```
┌─────────────────┐
│                 │
│ Diagnosis       │
│            ┌─────────────────┐
│            │                 │
└────────────│                 │
             │ Prognosis       │
             │                 │
             └─────────────────┘
```

After the diagnosis is *established*, the physician now consults his medical texts to learn the biologic behavior of this *disease*.

How much pain? How much suffering? How rapidly will the disease progress? What would be the degree of disability? What would be the probability of crippling deformities? Next, he consults medical texts to learn what results can be expected by treatment with various drugs. This is where the real trouble for patient begins.

Of course, statistics in medical texts were derived by studies conducted with the double-blind cross-over method of testing the efficacy of drugs. It means that in these studies, both the physician and the patient were kept in the blind as to the nature of the treatment. In these drug studies, the researchers bend over backwards to assure that the patient does not know what is being done to his biology. The study design mandates that the patient be systematically, diligently, and unfailingly excluded from exerting any influence over his illness (this is wishful thinking, as we shall soon see).

Returning to our patient with rheumatoid arthritis, she should know that *all* drugs used for rheumatoid arthritis are designed to suppress symptoms. Drug therapy is not designed to reverse the tissue injury by recognizing and removing those factors which cause it. Steroids, when used for this condition, relieve symptoms initially, but the patient pays a formidable long-term cost (in truly life-threatening situations, steroids work well). Finally, she should recognize that her only true chance to recognize the factors which may be initiating or perpetuating tissue injury is through tests for food and mold allergy, environmental triggers, viral and other microbial infections, specific autoimmune dysfunctions, and stress factors.

If the patient with rheumatoid arthritis (an autoimmune disorder) does choose drugs as her primary therapy, she should do this as an informed person, and not as an unknowing captive, "boxed-in" in the prognosis box.

THE THIRD BOX OF BOXOSIS

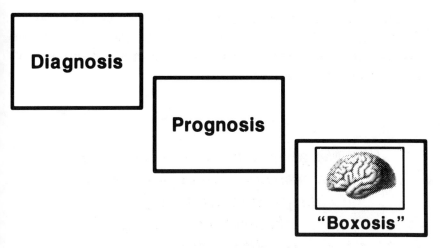

Brain Boxed Up In The Boxes   ALI

A journey through the boxes of diagnosis and prognosis now leads him to the final box. The patient is now ready to be incarcerated in the box of boxosis.

The massiveness of our medical edifices, the sheer aura of our high-tech, the regiments of *healthcare providers*, the intimidation of white coats, the weight of medical statistics, the *accumulated experience* of the physicians, the *Gods of peer review,* and the nods from all-knowing reimbursers, all join hands to assure submission of the patient. He now enters this final box of *boxosis*. He has no choice except to accept their verdict: the *drug of choice*.

The dogma of three D s has now delivered its promise. The patient has been effectively and totally excluded from the recovery process, the lip service about exercise and cholesterol-free diet notwithstanding.

Even the government now dictates in many circumstances the drug dose which the patient must take if his hospital stay is to be covered.

The incarceration of the patient's brain into our drug model is now completed. What patient has the courage to go up against all this? In the rare instance when he rebels against drugs or surgery, it is a *distraction* for us. We brand him as an eccentric or a *difficult patient*. We dismiss outright his own belief system, his own insights into the nature of his illness, his own strategies for recovery. We go on with our routine work of prescribing drugs.

A physician's first responsibility is to teach the masses not to take drugs.

Sir William Osler

I reiterate here what I wrote earlier in this volume. We can choose to consider nutritional medicine as a hoax. We can see environmental medicine as treatment of disease which does not exist. We can dismiss self-healing as a simple-minded and wishful pursuit. If we elect to do so, what alternatives to drugs do we have?

When the only tool one has is a hammer, everything looks like a nail to him.

Returning to the story of the young woman with the *disease* of rheumatoid arthritis, she is told to expect continued pain and tissue damage unless she accepts drug treatment. She is also advised of the possibility of advanced disease and crippling deformities. Self-regulation with nutritional and environmental concerns is not considered as an option. Should she choose to consider it, she is branded as an eccentric who does not see the dangers of the *untried methods.*

In the drug mode, the Physicians Desk Reference (PDR) is our bible. It is the final arbiter.

> *PDR does not contain a single entry of a*
> *drug which does not have side-effects*
> *but those are accepted as dangers*
> *of "tried" methods.*

Cancer and Boxosis

If our woman with rheumatoid arthritis was to develop a cancer, the box of boxosis becomes a box of tyranny. The stage is now set for us physicians to put limits on how long she should live. All this, of course, is *validated* by our statistics. Cancer prognosis becomes a pronouncement for death.

Cancer requires prompt and precise diagnosis. It calls for experienced hands to expeditiously remove the tumor. At times it requires adjunct therapy such as radiotherapy and chemotherapy. Most important of all, it requires the patient to know that:

Cancer statistics for survival are of limited relevance to her.

How are the statistics of survival for patients with cancer derived? Every patient with cancer must seek an answer to this most crucial of all questions?

*No two cancers are ever the same just as
no two cancer patients are the same.*

During the last 25 years of my work as a pathologist, I have personally studied more than 20,000 cancers. I do not know of any two cancers which were identical in their morphology, in their size and mode of spread, in the extent of invasion of the surrounding tissues, and which occurred in two individuals who were identical in their biologic make-up, in their life circumstances, in their hopes and spirits, and in their ability and willingness to fight their cancer. Talk to some senior pathologist during some cocktail hour, catch him off- guard, and ask him if he ever saw two identical cancers in two identical individuals. The answer will be the same. Now reflect on it for a few moments. What does it say about our cancer statistics ?

*Understanding the biology of tumors is
different from understanding the
biology of people who have
to carry those tumors.*

We understand some aspects of the biology of most tumors. Some cancers are anaplastic (undifferentiated) tumors. Such tumors are disorderly in appearance and strike early with distant spread (metastasis). Other cancers are well-differentiated. These tumors look orderly and imitate the tissue of their origin; their growth is slow and their potential for spread limited. These morphologic patterns of neoplasms are well-recognized.

What we understand poorly is the biology of tissues which serve as hosts to these tumors. This is where our problems begin.

We lump cancers of similar types together, ignore totally the host immune and nutritional factors, systematically exclude any role that a patient's own healing powers can play in his recovery, use ever-changing combinations of treatment methods, and then compute our survival numbers. We are a numerical people. We are now ready to live by these numbers. When challenged, we are ready to defend our numbers, fiercely when called upon to do so.

Dismissing the Anecdotal

When a patient with cancer does not follow our script, we are ingenious in inventing explanations for the bizzare behavior of patients and their tumors. We call the patients *exceptional*. We designate their tumors as *atypical*. When these explanations do not hold up, we have the old reliable *anecdotal*. This never fails. The surest strategy to discredit clinical observations which do not fit into the molds of diseases described in medical texts is to label it as *anecdotal*. The anecdotal, we are told over and over again in medical schools, is the crutch of the feeble-minded. The anecdotal has no place in the serious medical community. It is always a fatal blow to any defense one can marshall for self-regulation.

And so it is that these *rare* cases of control over cancer become *rarer* each time we deny their existence.

Young physicians, fresh from their residency training, are brimming with statistics. They see cancer as a mechanical problem to be approached with surgery, or as a problem of mutant cells to be destroyed with radiotherapy or chemotherapy. They see it a war of numbers in which the score is kept in *survival figures.* Medical students do not always start out that way. Most of them do have some sense of the complexity of the healing processes. They are not committed to the mechanics of medicine. It is the process of medical education which *sanitizes* them. The subjects of healing energy, holistic relatedness of human biology, love and hope, prayer, and self-regulation are taboo subjects.

Most older physicians who work with cancer patients eventually recognize that there is more to this problem than surgery, with or without radiotherapy and chemotherapy. This is where things go wrong: The older physicians do not wish to engage their younger colleagues and risk being regarded as *old-timers*, behind times in our thinking. And so it is that we perpetuate this myth of "anecdotal information". Little do we recognize that almost all truly great medical discoveries and insights came to us because one of us refused to dismiss as anecdotal a patient who did not fit into our textual models of disease.

Clinical observations made by Hippocrates, Galen, Memonedes, Semmelweis, Pasteur, Pare, Hunter and Osler, all were anecdotal in nature.

We may not be able to understand and quantify the energy of love and prayer for many decades, but we must not deny it just because we cannot measure it.

There are dimensions of healing for patients with cancer which we do not understand. There are aspects of healing energy which we may not know for many decades, even centuries. The technology which will allow us to measure such healing energy may not be forthcoming for many decades. There are just so many things in this area which simply cannot be denied. My thoughts do not represent mere conjecture or wishful thinking. It is a matter of many personal observations.

Two friends with melanoma in the liver

Sometime ago, I diagnosed malignant melanoma in a needle aspiration biopsy of a liver mass, the size of a golf ball. The patient was a friend of Talat, my wife. Her husband is one of my colleagues. The day after diagnosis, I spoke to him. He told me she knew it was time for her to go. She was prepared for it. She never left the hospital. She died within a period of three weeks.

Within several months of this, I diagnosed malignant melanoma in a needle aspiration biopsy of another liver mass, again the size of a golf ball. This patient, also a friend of Talat and the wife of one of my colleagues, is alive and free of tumor, five years after the diagnosis at the time of this writing.

After making the diagnosis, I went to see the second patient.

"I have confidence in you," I had said, not knowing what else to say.
"I am going to lick it," she replied.

She underwent removal of the right lobe of her liver at the Sloane Kettering Hospital in New York.

Melanoma is a lethal cancer. Once it has metastasized to

the liver, it is considered terminal. It is not considered amenable to surgery. Chemotherapy and radiotherapy are not effective. Self-healing is not acceptable to classical medicine.

Melanoma is a highly malignant tumor. Still it is not so malignant that she could not *lick* it. Is she an exceptional patient? A subject matter of an anecdote? A statistical anomaly? An oddity? A tribute to a surgeon's manual dexterity? A triumph of modern medicine? I do not know how much truth there might be in any of these suppositions. I do know how I see her. She is a heroine who won against all odds, and against all our pronouncements?

Two brothers with prostate cancer

Two bothers developed cancer of the prostate gland within a period of some months. At the time of diagnosis, the cancer in the first brother was limited to tissues in close vicinity of the gland. He died of his cancer within two years. At the time of diagnosis, the cancer in the second brother had already spread extensively to his bones. He lived for eleven years after the diagnosis. He suffered from other diseases, and it was not clear what role his cancer played in his death.

Why did one brother who would have been expected to live longer, die so soon? Why did the second brother who should have died sooner, live longer?

Cancers do not read medical texts.

As far as I know, cancers do not read our medical texts. They do not seem to have any compulsion to follow the mandates of our books, especially when we wrote our books without consulting them. Patients with cancer should know that medical texts about cancer are written by writers who do not know, or choose to ignore, the role of self-healing in treatment and control of cancer.

The brother who lived longer did so because he lived a better life. I know some of the circumstances of these two cases. I did not prove this with a double-blind cross-over study. It is just a simple *non-scientific* sense that I have.

36 women with breast cancer who were left out

Spiegel and his colleagues published an important paper last year in the prestigious British journal the *Lancet* (1989. Vol II: 888). They studied the effect on survival times of psychological intervention with supportive group therapy and self-hypnosis for pain in 86 patients with metastatic breast cancer. Fifty patients comprised the study group and the remaining 36 patients served as the control group. Both groups received similar oncological care. The patients in the study group lived twice as long as those in the control group (mean of 36.6 months vs mean of 18.9 months).

Spiegel, et al write, "We started with the belief that positive psychological and symptomatic effects could occur without affecting the course of the disease; we expected to improve the quality of life without affecting its quantity -------- We intended, in particular, to examine the often overstated claims made by those who teach cancer patients that the right mental attitude will help to conquer the disease ------ Future studies of the impact of psychological intervention on medical illness might profitably examine variables such as compliance, health habits, diet, and immune and neuroendocrine function."

When I read this paper, my thoughts went to the unfortunate 36 women in the control group who lost out on some important time of their lives. Why did it happen? So that we can satisfy our *scientific* curiosity? Or that we may meet some scientific standards of medical research? Or so that we can build a control group to satisfy the editors of some medical journal and get the paper published? I wondered which one of these reasons would be acceptable to any of those 36 women.

Is this study going to convert some medical statisticians into proponents of self-regulation? I doubt that.

What makes this subject so sad is that this is not the first study which has documented the efficacy of self-healing in the treatment and control of cancer. Spiegel, et al write, "Many studies have demonstrated positive psychological effects of group therapy in cancer patients, including improvements in mood, adjustment, and pain ------- In general, patients who receive psychotherapy survived longer." See appendix for additional references.

Patients with unresectable cancers (n= 204) were followed to determine the length of survival. -------- indicates that social and psychological factors individually or in combination do not influence the length of survival or the time of relapse.

New England Journal of Medicine
1985;312:1551-5

This study is quoted often by those who find the very idea of self-regulation offensive (I am always at a loss whenever I hear a physician expressing his anger on this subject). This study requires some comments.

The main group of patients in this study had what the investigators regarded as "unresectable cancers". They write, "The expected mean survival for patients in these categories is less than one year." For the patients in this study, the above two statements (in researcher's own words) must have meant simple and straight-forward death pronouncements. Nothing was offered to these patients. It is clear from this report that no hope was held out for these patients. The patients must have understood this.

Questionnaire Research

This study belongs to what I call *questionnaire research*. In this research model, the researcher makes no attempt to influence the outcome. That is exactly what was done in this study. After pronouncing imminent death to the patients in the study, the researchers limited themselves to studying how faithful to their script their patients were going to be till they died.

Twenty nine patients elected not to be faithful to the script chosen by the researchers.

Referring to 29 patients in this study, the authors of this report write, "have remained alive for 25 or more months since the diagnosis." Here was an opportunity to try to learn from these 29 patients something about why some people live longer with their cancers while others do not. No such attempts was made.

Researchers avoided the area of how their patients with *unresectable cancers* coped with their tumors because it would have been difficult to measure, considered as mysticism, and probably resulted in rejection of the paper.

Bad numbers are driving good sense out of our work as physicians.

There was a time the physician *cared* for his patient. The patient compensated his physician directly. Numbers were of small significance.

Now we physicians are *providers* in the healthcare business. We are numbers-driven. Our work is measured by numbers. We are compensated by numbers. We are punished if the numbers are not *right*. We all know young and old patients who died *but did not have to. But they died with right numbers.* That is acceptable because the *numbers* fitted the template of the *prevailing medical standards.*

There is some factor between a patient and his cancer that determines the outcome.

Verna Atkins, M.D.
Staff pathologist, Holy Name Hospital.

Dr. Atkins spoke the above words as she asked Evalynne

Braun, M.D., my associate pathologist, and I to review the biopsy of a vaginal lesion of Mary K. Mary underwent resection of an advanced rectal cancer in 1981. The cancer was aggressive in its morphology (microscopic appearance), had penetrated through the wall of rectum, and involved the regional lymph nodes. Nine years later, she developed a second cancer in her uterus which was removed with hysterectomy. There was no evidence of the first cancer at surgery. Now she had returned with a recurrence of the second uterine cancer. She would have been expected to die of her first cancer, but she didn't.

Mary is not unique in this. I have a large file of case histories like this. So what is this *factor* which allows some cancer patients to win?

Prognosis or pronouncement?

What would happen if patients with cancer were treated, but were given no prognosis?

Drs. Braun and Atkins and I talked about it one day as we reviewed some cancer cases. An 88 years old woman had a large neck cancer removed four years previously. The cancer had already spread to lymph nodes. She was not expected to live. Now she returned four years later with a recurrent cancer.

She was active and alert and not very concerned about extensive surgery which was now being planned. A man returned with a recurrent lung cancer several years after he had been *written off* as terminal. There were other cases like that.

How did we physicians get so caught up in this game of *survival figures?* How are these survival figures derived? What do they really represent? How did we learn to turn these cold numbers of dubious value into firm pronouncements of death? How do we become so prescient about life and death?

I believe a time will come when the patients will accept from us physicians the diagnoses of cancer, but will say, "No, thank you." to our pronouncement of prognosis and death. Or perhaps we physicians will realize this sooner than our patients, and will not have to develop strategies for "coping" with defiant patients.

A Statistician or a Sufi?

Who should a person with cancer listen to? A statistician of medicine or a Sufi of molecular medicine? The statistician will number his days; the Sufi will teach him what to do with those days and many more. He will teach him something about Dr. Atkin's *factor.*

Diagnosis of cancer must be precise. Mapping out the tissues involved with cancer must be accurate. Surgery, chemotherapy and radiotherapy, in whatever combinations are most effective for the given cancer, must be undertaken promptly and skillfully. There is no room for error in all this. Sometimes the patient needs time before he is ready for all this. This is the way it should be. There is no valid scientific reason why a person cannot take whatever time he feels is necessary for making his decision to proceed with treatment.

The real battle with cancer begins, in my judgement, after all these logistical things have been done. That is when the patient has a choice.

He can listen to a medical statistician and let him set limits on how long he can live.

or

*He can listen to a Sufi of molecular medicine
and learn how molecular injury begins,
how it threatens the integrity of
molecular systems, and how
these molecular systems
can be repaired.*

Surgery, with or without radiotherapy and chemotherapy, damages the immune system, often severely. A patient with cancer should know that a damaged immune system can be repaired with protocols of nutritional medicine, environmental medicine, medicine of self-healing, and medicine of fitness. Of these, medicine of self-healing, it seems to me, is the single most valuable resource.

We physicians often are troubled by these ideas. Why ?

First, because we physicians are incarcerated in our own box of *boxosis of the double-blind.* Since self-healing cannot be double-blinded, we simply deny it.

Second, we make the sad error of looking at self-healing as a threat to our roles as the *healers*. It is sad because we physicians never heal any patients. What we do well is to remove some of the impediments in the way of healing. We can do the same in the theatre of self-healing as we do in the operating theatres (in Mayo hospital, Lahore where I began my surgical training, the east wing of the operating suites is still called the *East Theatre*).

Third, we physicians consider ourselves scientists. We consider self-healing as mysticism. We are taught that the surest way to jeopardize our standing as scientists is to be associated with mystics. I will let you in on a secret: most experienced physicians are *closet mystics*. How can one we through life seeing patients live who are expected to die, and watch people die who should have lived, and not wonder? How can we not become a mystics?

The Aztecs appease their God QuetzalcoatL

I will let you in on another secret. We older physicians live in fear of being branded *old-timers* by our younger colleagues. Our defense: total, utter, and unfaltering submission to the *Gods of double-blind cross-over*. The Aztecs sacrificed their young with perfect bodies and best minds to appease their God, Quetzalcoatl. We older physicians sacrifice our most treasured clinical observations to appease our *God of the double-blind.*

There is the apocryphal story of a
statistician who drowned in a
stream with an average
depth of two feet.

There is another apocryphal story of a patient who faced dangerous surgery. He consulted a second surgeon for a second opinion.

"What are my chances of living through this surgery,doc?"
"One hundred percent," replied the surgeon.
"But doc, I heard nine out of ten patients die with this operation. How do you know I will live?"
"Yes, that is true," answered the surgeon, "but all nine patients who went before you died. You are the tenth patient. Statistically, you must live."

And what is a second opinion?
One opinion for which the patient pays twice.

A Mother's Love. Unproven? Inappropriate?

Mary consulted me for multiple myeloma, a variant of bone marrow cancer. She was first diagnosed two years previously and given chemotherapy. Now she saw me for a recurrence. She had strong feelings against additional chemotherapy which her oncologist was advising. I recommended that it was a sound approach for this type of cancer (I do not recommend chemotherapy for all cancers. Indeed, there have been times when I wondered if the indication of chemotherapy for a patient had been his presence in the oncologist's office.)

Politely, but firmly, Mary declined my recommendation (this is always acceptable to me).

Some weeks later, she attended one of my *auto-regulation* workshops for patients and decided to learn and practice it. She is a very intuitive person. Within a few days she was able to perceive the energy which is the essence of *auto-regulation.* One day she called Talat and related to her with excitement how she was able to direct the *pulses* and do *limbic breathing.* She then told her she had decided to accept chemotherapy. So now she is doing it because she is listening to her *limbic voice, I thought.* This is, in my judgement, the way it should be. Next, she told Talat how her insurance carrier had refused to reimburse her for her *auto-regulation* training session, even after it was explained *auto-regulation* is a specialized form of self-regulation for disease prevention and treatment.

I do not know if Orwell ever thought of the day when the

government statisticians will declare a mother's affection for her child unproven, and hence inappropriate. Unindicated? Non-reimbursable? To my knowledge, nobody has ever done a controlled study to prove that a mother's love is beneficial for the child. How would a child know when he is in the study group and must accept his mother as his mother, and when he is in the control group and must not accept his mother as his mother?

NOTION OF IRREVERSIBILITY

The single largest hurdle in the way of self-regulation and healing is what Norman Cousins has called the *notion of irreversibility.*

In his book, the *Healing Heart,* Cousins wrote the story of his massive heart attack and his recovery. At one point his physicians wanted him to undergo coronary angiography, as a prelude to bypass surgery. Cousins was resistant to this idea.This is how he relates his conversation with his physician, Dr. Shine.

"What would you like me to do?" I asked.
"I think you ought to go back to hospital and have an

angiogram. That way we can determine exactly where the blockage is, how serious is it, and how best to correct it."

"I realized that this meant bypass surgery. Since the blockage was also established, the angiogram would serve as the road map for the surgeon.

"Isn't it possible that the condition of my arteries has improved along with the general improvement of everything else?" I asked.

"The heart itself has been undergoing a healing experience," he said, *"but that process does not extend to the coronary arteries."*

Why not I wondered when I first read *The Healing Heart?* This is a remarkable statement to come from a physician. In my study and practice of pathology of over thirty years, I have never come across any healing phenomenon within the human frame which would support such a contention. Indeed, recent research has shown clearly that established plaque in coronary arteries can be cleared without surgical intervention.

Cousins's story becomes more illuminating. He continues,

"When the walls of the arteries are lined by accumulated plaque, you have to contend with ongoing coronary artery disease."

"Hasn't there been some research," I asked, *" showing that, when the level of cholesterol in the blood is reduced and stays reduced over a period of time, the arteries widen? What about the work of Lester Morrison? How about the evidence assembled*

by Dr. Castelli of NIH?"

"The most comprehensible studies on the subject have been carried out by David Blankenhorn, of USC," Dr. Shine replied. "These studies showed that the femoral arteries in human beings could be freed of blockage to some extent, but there was no corresponding improvement in the coronary arteries. The evidence you cite is interesting, but not yet conclusive."

There is another remarkable statement by a physician. The femoral arteries can be freed of blockage but not the coronary arteries. Why not? What distinguishes the coronary arteries from the femoral arteries so much that one set of arteries can be freed and not the other? What kind of evidence could a physician possibly marshall to support such a view? I have often wondered about our convictions of what constitutes conclusive evidence in medicine. Cousins continues,

"Then you don't think the program I am on will have the effect of bringing more oxygen to the heart?"

"I wish I could encourage you to believe you have reversed the problem in your coronary arteries," he said, "but this is not what accumulated experience says will happen."

Here is the third remarkable statement of a physician. The *accumulated experience* here refers to the experience of physicians with patients who had been convinced that their (patient's) own healing powers were irrelevant to their recovery from illness. The *accumulated experience* here also refers to the double-blind cross-over model of research in clinical medicine.

Double-blind, by definition, means that both the patient and the physician were kept blind to the nature of treatment used. How can such *accumulated experience* be considered relevant to somebody yearning for self-regulation and healing? Self-regulation, by definition, cannot be blinded. Let us continue with Cousins's story.

As Dr. Shine spoke, I thought to myself, "Here we go again." I felt a surge of energy and couldn't suppress a smile.

Dr. Shine asked whether he had said anything funny. I replied that he hadn't; it was just that the notion of irreversibility had touched off something deep inside me. That was the concept that had been used to describe the condition, 17 years earlier, that I wrote about in Anatomy of an Illness.

One last comment about the immune-collagen disease which had afflicted Cousins 17 years before his heart attack. During my years of work in diagnostic pathology, I have examined thousands of biopsies of patients with various forms of so-called collagen and autoimmune disorders. Except when we can identify the molecules which cause such disorders (allergy, chemical sensitivity, and some viral and bacterial organisms), all these disease names are but mere diagnostic labels. Unfortunately many of these individuals are told they have *irreversible* disorders. They are then prescribed steroids and other immuno-suppressant drugs. Many who escape, or steadfastly refuse such prognostications (and therapies which follow) do go on to *reverse* their illness, just as Norman Cousins did his.

The Blessed Double-blind cross-over

A visiting professor in our hospital was lecturing on the care of patients with heart attacks after they leave the hospital. At one point, he referred to the work of a west coast group of physicians who conducted a study on the effects of stress management on recovery from heart attacks. They had reported substantial clinical benefits compared with the patients in the control group (who were not given such therapy). One of the criteria they used was the patient's own assessment of the benefits of the stress reduction program. The speaker was chagrined with this element of self-appraisal. He lamented the lack of scientific validity in a study model in which the patients were required to evaluate the efficacy of treatment (the patients in this study evidently could not have been blinded to the fact that they were being trained to manage their stress). At one point, the speaker got so frustrated with this aspect of this study that he blurted out,

"The patients felt better. But what does that mean ?"

It does matter. It matters a whole lot to the patient. I wondered if he really understood what his words meant.

Bad statistics are driving good sense out of a physician's work. We physicians do get confused about our goals when we talk of science in medicine. Why do patients see us? So that *we* can feel good about *our* work? Or celebrate *our* science? Or bask in the glory of *our* blessed double-blind cross-over? Patients consult us so we can help *them* feel better, relieve their suffering, and reverse their diseases. They compensate us for our services with this hope. I do not see any patients who are concerned with double-blind cross-over. Patients want to feel better, double-blind or no double-blind.

The real issue in clinical medicine is outcome. In the treatment of acute disease with potent (and toxic) drugs, as I indicated earlier, double-blind cross-over method is a useful model for investigation. In the treatment of chronic disorders with protocols of nutritional medicine, environmental medicine, and medicine of self-healing, our goals should be gradual restoration of health and not mere symptom suppression. These protocols produce their desired results at a slower rate than are seen with drugs. These modes of treatment cannot be blinded. The only model for investigation in this context is that based on clinical outcomes with different treatment plans.

When double-blind blinds no one.

There is an amusing aspect of this, our *blessed* double-blind cross-over model of research. It is seldom spoken about in polite medical company. From personal experience, I know that no physician and patient can be kept in the blind as to the nature of the treatment for any significant length of time (I assume that both the physician and the patient have some measure of curiosity and intellect). Whenever I have discussed this subject (at a cocktail hour) with any of my colleagues in clinical research, they readily admitted to me that they came to know the identity of the placebo and the drug within a very short time of starting the study. The same held for the patient. Notwithstanding, they continued with the study (and the facade of double-blind). How else do you publish the results? How else do you get a drug approved by FDA?

The researcher and the patient find out the true identity of the drug and the placebo in several predictable ways. First is the intended chemical effect of the drug on the way a patient feels. From a purely theoretical perspective, the only way the two can be confused for any length of time is if the drug does not have any effect at all. If it does, the drug will exert its chemical effect and will be readily recognized by that.

The second clue to the identity of the drug is the effect of the drug on the laboratory tests. Patients in research studies undergo extensive testing; drugs change the test results while the placebo does not. It amuses me to read about research studies comparing highly toxic drugs (which rapidly suppress bone marrow) with the placebo. Recent study of DDI (a highly toxic drug) for AIDS is a case in point. All patients quickly developed serious marrow depression and anemia; predictably, the placebo group did not develop this complication. The patients in the drug group and health professionals knew they had become more anemic (due to the drug use). Those in the placebo group knew they had not suffered from any chemical consequences of DDI. While some researchers extolled the value of this study, others pronounced the study data worthless.

How can such studies ever be considered *blinded*?

The informed consent forms which patients sign for entry into research studies outline in great detail all possible adverse effects of the drug. The patients are well-sensitized to the risks involved and about what to look for. And they do.

Finally, physicians and patients have an intuitive sense of what works for them and what does not. Placebos do not carry the chemical effects of drugs, are benign in usage, and are intuitively distinguished from the drugs by both the physician and the patient.

In closing, I should add a comment about one other aspect of double-blind. In the research treatment of chronic disorders, patient almost *never* do *only* what their physicians tell them to do. They always add to that treatment many aspects of nutrition, environmental changes, and stress management in *varying* degrees. It is simply not possible to eliminate all other variables for the duration of the study. The statistics obtained with such studies are just that, mere statistics. They have only limited relevance to a given patient with a given disease.

Patients with cancer and severe autoimmune disorders must not let anyone set limits on how long they are going to live based on any statistics.

Don't deny the diagnosis, just defy the verdict which is supposed to go with it.

Norman Cousins

MASK OF ANGER

Chronic anger, in my experience, is one of the foremost risk factors for chronic illness. It is also one of the foremost factors in recovery from chronic illness. In my work with *auto-regulation,* it clearly has been the single most important hurdle in the way of progress with self-healing. The *cortical monkey* does its best work through anger. In the chapter on **Ten Lessons Learned from Patients,** I wrote that psychosomatic and somatopsychic models of disease are artifacts of our thinking. Diseases are burdens on biology. Chronic anger is a heavy burden on biology.

Biology of Anger

The ancients seemed to know the workings of anger intuitively. We need technology to gain insights into the biology of anger. The biology of anger, in essence, is the biology of accelerated aging process. It is a state of spinning biologic wheels, unwittingly and needlessly, a condition of *biologic burnout*.

Chronic anger regularly expresses itself as:

- increased vaso-motor tone
    (tight arteries impeding free flow of blood)

- Quickened heart rate
    (tired heart pushing blood through tight arteries)

- Higher respiratory rate
    (increased oxidative molecular damage)

- increased electromyo-potentials
    (muscle fibers fatigued by unrecognized spasms)

- Higher frequency of brain waves
    (sending stress signals to all tissues)

- Irregular motility of bowel musculature with spasms
    (turbulence in bowel with altered ecology)

- Increased catabolism
    (accelerated tissue wear and tear)

I have repeatedly observed all these changes in patients with high residue of chronic anger. These patho-physiologic changes can be readily documented with appropriate electromagnetic technology.

Anger, the silent monkey

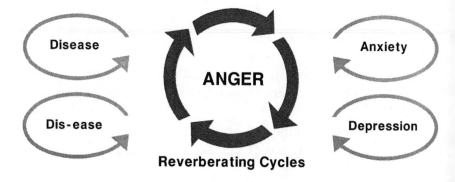

Reverberating Cycles

Chronic anger is one of the foremost burdens on an

individual's biology.

Anger is a molecular lesion.

Hate is a molecular lesion, and so is pain and suffering.

Love is a molecular event.

Hope is a molecular event. Indeed, life is an uninterrupted sequence of molecular events.

Psychosomatic and somatopsychic models of disease are artifacts of our thinking. This is a critically important point, and I repeat it several times in this volume and in the companion volume *The Pheasant and Suffering in Illness.*

Pathologists, immunologists, and biologists know that the adverse molecular and electro-magnetic events unleashed by *bad feelings* of anger are *identical* to those triggered by stress, of an excess of acid in the stomach, a bowel spasm, choking of tissues by tight arteries, or tissues hurt by a virus.

It is not possible in clinical practice to clearly distinguish between molecular events which are initiated by anger from those which are caused by other types of biologic insults to human tissues.

What sets the *cortical monkey* of chronic anger apart from

other monkeys is its silent and unforgiving nature. It beats up on the unsuspecting tissues, ceaselessly and mercilessly. The victims, in my experience, have generally been very intelligent individuals, often in professions of health, education and business.

I show in a schematic fashion in the preceding illustration how the reverberating cycles of anxiety, depression, dis-ease, and disease continuously feed the larger central cycle of anger. Failure to resolve chronic anger makes complete recovery unlikely in most patients. This schema is also intended to provide a rationale for integrating methods of self-regulation with treatment protocols of nutritional and environmental medicines.

Susan's Story

Susan was a professor in a local college for many years before she retired. She is a very pleasant person, always courteous and with a smile on her face. Several years before she saw me, she had both breasts removed for two separate cancers, the second operation following the first one within several months. She had been free of cancer ever since.

Susan consulted me for allergy and recurring episodes of headache, worse at the time of ovulation. She spoke confidently about how she could always tell when she ovulated even though she had reached menopause several years earlier.

One of the events she related to me during her initial visit was about a difficult experience she had with an oncologist who tried to *force* chemotherapy on her because he suspected metastatic cancer in her spine. This proved to be a false alarm.

" I have never been well since then," she said.

I did not recognize the pivotal role of this event in her chronic illness until much later.

She had heard of my work with nutrition and self-regulation. After attending an *auto-regulation* seminar, she seemed extremely receptive to my treatment protocols of allergy, nutrition, and *auto-regulation*. Following diagnostic testing, I initiated my treatment protocols. Initially, she made satisfactory progress.

Blood drops falling out of a gem.

Limbic image is a term I use for the image a person sees during *auto-regulation* which he does not understand and which his thinking *cortical mind* would not have created in ordinary circumstances. I regard such an image as an important milestone in progress in *auto-regulation*.

Susan made some progress with *auto-regulation* initially. During one period of *auto-regulation* with me, she suddenly became agitated and angry. She said, "I saw a beautiful gem with gorgeous colors. I was totally captivated by its beauty and then suddenly I see blood drops coming out of it. That frightened me. The blood drops brought back *that hos*pital memory."

I never saw Susan again.

There is an ancient story which translated into the contemporary vernacular goes something like this:

A man suffered from a chronic illness. He saw many physicians and tried different medicines. Nothing worked. Finally, he went to see a sage of his time. The sage listened to his sad story and advised him to go out to the fields each morning, face the rising sun, look to the heavens, raise his hands and say, " Lord, fill me with thy spirits." He agreed to do so.

Next morning, he went out to the fields and did exactly what the sage had asked him to do. Nothing happened. He did the same the next morning, and the next morning. Nothing happened. He returned to the sage and told him about this. The sage again listened to the man and asked him to repeat the same words in a much louder voice.

Next morning the man went out to the fields and shouted in a loud voice, Lord, fill me with thy spirit."

There was a loud thunder, and then a heavy voice came,

"Damn it, I do. But you leak."

MASK OF FEAR OF SUFFERING

No one chooses a devastating illness to learn about the human spirit and human capacity for endurance. Still, chronic unremitting suffering is a great teacher. Some of my patients could (and I hope will) write their inspiring, and heart-rending stories of human capacity for absorbing severe and prolonged biologic punishments, sustaining hope against all odds, and finally emerging out of their illnesses with unbroken spirits. Bonnie and Jackie are two of many such individuals whom I have had the privilege to treat.

Bonnie's Story

Bonnie has a long history of life-threatening and incapacitating depression. For years she had suffered from daily headaches and frequent abdominal *migraine* attacks among other symptoms of depression. She received the standard psychiatric care with drugs and psychotherapy. When the situation got out of control, she was hospitalized.

Bonnie also suffers from inhalant allergy and sensitivity to perfumes, formaldehyde and some other chemicals. Blood tests for volatile hydrocarbons showed raised levels of several solvents and other hydrocarbons. She responded well to allergy and nutritional protocols. One particular item which proved to be very helpful was replacement of a gas cooker with an electric one. Her suffering from depression, however, continued with some abatement.

Bonnie did not tolerate her medication well. That is how she became interested in the possibility of self-regulation for control of her depression symptoms.

After considerable initial difficulties and many hours of work with tapes, she finally learned well the methods of *directed pulses, limbic breathing,* and *tissue sensing.* She was then able to regularly and predictably dissolve her headaches and other symptoms of depression with *auto-regulation.*

Still, she continued to suffer from depression, at times intensely. I was puzzled why she did not make more progress. I knew she practiced *auto-regulation* regularly and effectively. One day I asked her if she had some thoughts about why she was not able to dissolve *all* her suffering caused by depression. She thought for a while and then replied,

"I can dissolve most of my suffering with auto-reg, but then I become very scared that all my suffering will come back. I think it is this fear of suffering which brings back my suffering."

Shapes of suffering

Human suffering has three shapes: a shape of remembered suffering, a shape of suffering of the *moment*, and a shape of the feared future suffering.

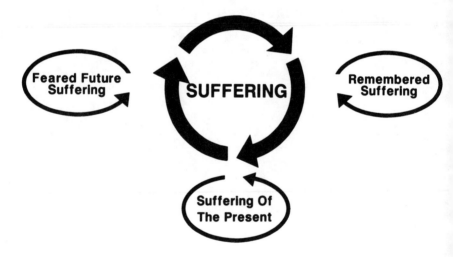

For most patients in captivity of chronic unremitting

suffering, the suffering of the *moment* is far less intimidating than the remembered suffering or the feared future suffering. It is far easier for them to learn how to obtain relief from the suffering of the moment than it is to dissipate the load of the remembered pain and suffering, or to dispel the fear of the feared future suffering.

The *cortical monkey* of fear is a tenacious creature, forever leaping back into the scene. The anomaly of brain chemistry which sets Bonnie up for suffering has not been reversed. So she still suffers. The difference now is that even in periods of intense suffering, she can see the way out. She does pull herself out of her deep hole of depression. She has learned to dissolve the fear.

Jackie's Story

As a teenager, Jackie suffered from nasal and sinus allergy which was treated with various drugs. For throat infections and "colds", she received multiple courses of antibiotics. In time she recognized her sensitivity to several foods.

Jackie grew up to be, in the words of her husband, a woman of "great energy". She had a happy marriage and stable family life with her children. She did not have "much stress problem".

In her late thirties she developed sensitivity to tobacco smoke, perfumes and formaldehyde. These problems did not interfere with her very active life.

One day she cleaned her basement and collected a lot of dust from the crevices in the walls. This is when, again in the words of her husband "her whole life came crashing down". Within weeks, she suffered from severe and disabling fatigue, rapidly lost weight, developed painful spasms of tongue and throat (sometimes with visible torsion of her tongue), saw spontaneous bruises on her arms and legs, and noticed irregularity of menstruation. She underwent exhaustive diagnostic work-up at two university hospitals in New York city. An ESR test showed abnormal results.

Ousted from her home.

Jackie was compelled to leave her house. She moved to her mother's apartment. That is where she still lives, more than three years after her collapse. All through this ordeal, her husband has been most supportive. There is another hero of mine.

I was one of over ten physicians she consulted. Her micro-Elisa tests showed multiple mold, pollen and food allergies. It was obvious that the cause of her devastating illness was a large exposure to some chemical.

Our search for the causative chemical turned out to be exasperating, time-consuming, and very expensive. We undertook extensive environmental surveys of the air in various parts of her house and the soil around the basement walls. We called in special laboratory personnel to conduct these tests. Finally, we succeeded in pinning down the poison.

The chemical villain

The chemical villain turned out to be Chlordane, an insecticide which had been drilled into the soil around the basement walls some years ago. Over the years, it rose to the ground level, found its way into the house through the cracks in the walls, accumulated in the dust in her basement, and laid there in darkness ready to strike. On the day of cleaning, she was hit in full force.

I performed a fat biopsy to document the presence of Chlordane and its breakdown products in Jackie's tissues. The analysis confirmed what we had clinically suspected: the levels of these chemicals in fatty tissues were high.

During the next two years, her progress was slow and intermittent. She continued to see one of her previous physicians for nutritional treatment and a second physician for some homeopathic remedies. I treated her for multiple allergies and taught her *auto-regulation*. She became adept at *auto-regulation*. Her skin bruises disappeared. She gained weight. Her energy level increased.

Inspite of all this progress, and despite many attempts to clear the house of Chlordane contamination, she was not able to return to her house.

One day she came to see me very frightened and in tears. She had gone out for dinner on a family occasion. She was exposed to tobacco smoke, perfumes, car exhaust, and some articles from her house. She developed severe reactions. Now she sat in my office, dejected and in despair.

> *"Dr. Ali, I am frightened for my life. I am losing everything I have worked so hard to get. I can't go through it all over again. This might end now. I will never really get out of it."*

Jackie pulled herself out of this episode just as she had fought her way out of so many others. She continues to make progress, though it is exasperatingly slow.

> *The first responsibility of a physician to a patient in despair with a severe chronic illness is to create and sustain hope.*

The first task is easy, the second, most demanding.

A small step in disease reversal.
A large leap in relief of symptoms.

Symptoms do not increase or decrease in a linear fashion with progression or reversal of disease. This is a significant issue.

Increasing intensity of disease does not cause a proportionate increase in the intensity of pain and suffering. Rather, it is similar to an exponential function; small increases in the disease process cause a disproportionately large increment in symptoms. The converse also occurs. Small reversals in the disease process afford disproportionately large measures of symptom relief.

Is suffering quantifiable ?

We physicians want to know the extent of suffering of our patients. Quantifying a patient's suffering in disease is a goal which has eluded us since the beginning of scientific method in medicine. Indeed, our disillusionment in this area is so profound that we are deeply suspicious of anybody who professes an interest in it. Among physicians, this is a taboo subject. Any reference to this subject is likely to be unceremoniously dismissed.

A patient's suffering may not be quantifiable for us physicians, and may not fit our *blessed* double-blind cross-over model of research, but *it is quantifiable* for the patient.

For a patient, the relationship between the extent of disease and the intensity of suffering inflicted by it has important implications in the field of self-regulation. It means that even a modest decrease in the molecular injury brought about with *s*elf-regulatory methods (*with appropriate nutritional and environmental protocols*) brings about a marked amelioration of symptoms. I illustrate this essential point in a schematic fashion with two diagrams.

In the first diagram, I show a simple linear mathematical relationship. This is the type of relationship that we are inclined to think of when we consider the relationship between molecular injury and suffering. In linear relationships, a change in one parameter is associated with an equivalent change in the other. Molecular injury and suffering, however, are biologic events, and simple linear relationships are not observed in biologic systems.

In the second diagram, I show a relationship which is seen in biologic systems. In scientific jargon, it is called a sigmoid relationship. In this relationship, a small change in one parameter is associated with a large change in the other. This is the basic nature of the relationship between molecular injury and suffering that I see in my patients. The relevance of this relationship to work with self-regulation is fundamental to success, both for the patient and the professional.

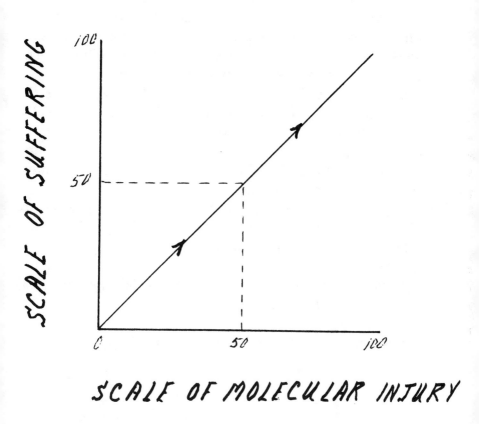

SCALE OF MOLECULAR INJURY

In the above diagram, I illustrate, in a schematic expression, the relationship between the extent of molecular injury and suffering from disease.

The scale of molecular injury along the horizontal axis

represents the extent of molecular and cellular injury (the intensity of disease). The scale of suffering along the vertical axis represents how much the patient suffers as a result of molecular injury. The intensity of the symptoms of disease is expressed along the vertical axis as a scale of suffering. The range of the two scales extends from a maximum of 100 to a minimum of zero. The value of one hundred represents the highest intensity of disease as well as suffering, while the value of zero represents absence of disease as well as suffering.

This diagram shows a *linear relationship*. In this direct relationship, each increase in the molecular injury is accompanied with an equivalent increase in the intensity of suffering. The zero point on the scale of suffering corresponds to the zero point on the scale of molecular injury; so do the corresponding points at 50 and 100 units. In clinical terms, this relationship requires that we reduce molecular injury by 50 % if we wish to control suffering by 50 %.

Now let us consider the *sigmoid* relationship.

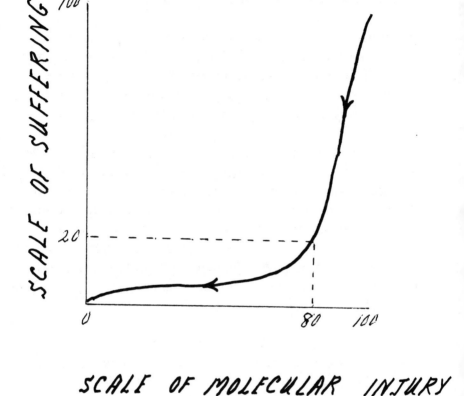

The diagram above shows a *sigmoid relationship*. In this relationship, a small change on the scale of molecular injury results in a disproportionately large change on the scale of suffering. Specifically, a 20 % reduction on the scale of molecular injury leads to an 80 % drop on the scale of suffering. In clinical context, it means that the patient can expect a very desirable 80 % relief in suffering if he can reduce molecular injury by a mere 20 %.

Which one of the two above relationships is true to life? Almost all biochemical relationships in human biology are of the *sigmoid* type. None are known to be of *linear* type. If we simply consider the probability, common sense tells us to look for a *sigmoid* relationship, and not a *linear* relationship.

To illustrate this critical point, I have chosen the 80/20 model which is well-known to us. From my own clinical experience, it seems to me that this proverbial and theoretical 20-80 ratio, if anything, is too conservative in the context of disease reversal and alleviation of suffering. Time and again, I see that relatively small reversals in molecular and electro-magnetic abnormalities obtained with *auto-regulation* (and protocols of nutritional and environmental medicine) are associated with large clinical benefits.

In my clinical work, the real number is in the range of 90/10 or 95/5. This implies that a mere reduction of 5-10 % in molecular injury can be expected to result in 90-95 % relief in suffering - a tremendous physiologic advantage for the patient.

Most clinicians will agree that patients receive relief of symptoms with treatment long before a significant change in molecular dynamics can be expected. I suspect that this or some mechanism similar to this explains how our patients control their asthma attacks or migraine pains with *auto-regulation* in short periods of time.

A New Medicine

Recently, I was a guest of Charles Carluccio, M.D. on his radio show *Human Medicine*. Charles started out by asking me how, in the best of possible worlds, patients with chronic health disorders could be treated?

In the best of the worlds, I thought, there will be a different medicine. It will be a new medicine with four faces: a face of Nutritional Medicine, a face of Environmental Medicine, a face of Medicine of Fitness, and a face of Medicine of Self-regulation and healing.

In the best of worlds, a patient will have access to a physician who knows the physiology of fitness, the pharmacology of nutrients, the chemistry of environmental pollutants, the immunology of allergy, the pathology of autoimmunity and biology of self-regulation and healing. This will be the beginning of a new molecular medicine. It will set medical thought free from the constraints of cellular pathology, just as Virchow's *cellular pathology* set us free from the constraints of the gross pathology of medieval and ancient times.

Charles asked me the expected question: Why are we physicians so resistent to such ideas?

This is a simple question. The answers are far from simple. There are the issues of the dogma of the three D s. There are the issues of the dogma of three boxes. There are the issues of our *blessed* double-blind cross-over. There are the issues of the prevailing standards of care. There are the issues of the government mandating how many drugs we must receive if our hospital bills are to be paid. Our medical reimbursement system is oriented toward procedures for testing and treating. It severely punishes those who are not eager to intervene with drugs, invasive instruments, or surgical scalpels. There are issues of economic punishment to the patients who want to be taught methods for self-regulation and healing, and to the physicians who want to teach these methods it to their patients.

I am an optimist. I believe this will all change. A growing number of us see the futility of trying to solve problems caused by chemicals with yet more chemicals. We recognize the error in blocking enzymes to relieve symptoms caused by blocked enzymes. As physicians become aware of these problems, so will their patients.

An increasing number of physicians and patients see the choice between drugs and non-drug molecular protocols. It is only a matter of time when they will begin to exercise their options. Some are doing so now.

*A great free nation must have freedom
of choice in matters of health
for its citizens.*

I started this book with healing energy and this is where I end it now.

Just as classical medicine moves from the model of cellular pathology to a model of molecular pathology, it will see the next peak on the horizon, a much taller peak of the energy medicine. It will be in this medicine that the healing energy from within, the energy of love, will find its clearest expression. This will call for yet another major realignment in medical thought, probably the most demanding of all changes that medicine has ever been called upon to make.

" *It's what Goethe said in Faust but which Lucas has dressed in modern idiom-the message that technology is not going to save us. Our computers, our tools, our machines are not enough. We have to rely on our intuition, our true being.*"

Joseph Campbell

Someday after mastering the winds, the waves, the tides and gravity, we shall harness for God the energies of love. And then for the second time in the history of the world man will have discovered fire.

Teilhard de Chardin

It seems improbable that man will ever fully understand the healing energy of love, or to be more precise the healing energy of God. Medical technology, itself an expression of God's energy, is beginning to allow us to measure some things about love, and then reproduce them. Measurements and reproducibility make up the language of science. One day, it seems, the men of medicine and the men of spirits will meet at some summit of union. The energy of love will have brought them together.

Section 7

Appendix

Reading Suggestions and References

The following books and tapes of Dr. Ali
are available from the

Institute of Preventive Medicine

320-Belleville Ave, Bloomfield, New Jersey, 07003
201-743-1151

Books

Nutrition for Life Span Molecules
The Dog and the Dis-ease Syndrome
The Pheasant and Suffering in Illness
Nutritional Medicine: Principles and Practice
The Altered Bowel Ecology Syndrome

Tapes

Tape 101: Basic Auto-reg training
Tape 103: Tissue Sensing Training
Tape 102: Limbic Breathing Training
Tape 21: The New Molecular Medicine
Tape 204: The Chronic Fatigue Syndrome
Tape 202: Auto-reg, Principles and Practice
Tape 203: The Altered Bowel Ecology Syndrome
Tape 22: Non-pharmacologic Management of Asthma

References for self-regulation

Ader, Robert, ed. Psychoneuroimmunology. New York: Academic Press, 1981.

Ader, R. and Cohen, N. Behaviorally Conditioned Immunosuppression and Murine Systemic Lupus Erythematosus. Science, 215:1534-1536, 1982.

Ader R, Cohen N. CNS-immune system interactions: conditioning phenomena, Behav Brain Sci 1985;8:379.

Ali, M. The Pheasant and Suffering in Illness. Bloomfield, New Jersey: Institute of Preventive Medicine. 1990

Ali, M. The Dog and the Dis-ease Syndrome. Bloomfield, New Jersey: Institute of Preventive Medicine. 1990.

Anand, B.K., G.S. Chhina, and B. Singh. Some aspects of electroencephalographic studies in yogis. Electroencep. Clin. Neurophysio., 1961, 13, 452-456.

Barber, T.X., et al., eds. Biofeedback and Self Control. A series of annuals beginning in 1971 in which leading articles in the field are republished each year. Chicago: Aldine-Atherton.

Bartrop RW, Luckhurst E, Lazarus L. Depressed lymphocyte function after bereavement. Lancet 1977;1:834.

Basmajian, John V. Muscles Alive: Their Functions Revealed by Electromyography. Baltimore: Williams & Wilkins, 1962.

Bennett, Hal, and Mike Samuels. The Well Body Book. New York: Random House, 1973.

Benson, Herbert, with Miriam Z. Klipper. The Relaxation Response. New York: Avon Books, 1976.

Benson, Herbert, with William Proctor. Your Maximum Mind. New York: Times Books, 1987.

Bensen, Herbert, and William Proctor. Beyond the Relaxation Response. New York: Berkley, 1985

Berk, L.S., Tan, S.A, Nehlsen-Cannarella, S.L., Napier, B.J., Lewis, J.E., Lee, J.W., Eby, W.C., & Fry W.F. (1988). Humor associated laughter decreases cortisol and increases spontaneous lymphocyte blastogenesis. Abstract presented at the American Federation for Clinical Research annual meeting.

Besedovsky HO, del Ray AE, Sorkin E. Immune-neuroendocrine interactions. J Immunol 1985;135:750s.

Black S, Humphrey JH, Niven JS. Inhibition of Mantoux reaction by direct suggestion under hypnosis. Br Med J 1962;1:1649.

Black, S. (1963). Inhibition of immediate-type hypersensitivity response by direct suggestion under hypnosis. British Medical Journal, 1, 925-929.

Black, S. (1963). Shift in dose-response curve of prausnitz-kustner reaction by direct suggestion under hypnosis. British Medical Journal, 1, 990-992.

Black, S., & Friedman, M. (1965). Adrenal function and the inhibition of allergic responses under hypnosis. British Medical Journal, 1, 562-567.

Black, S., & Humphrey, J. H., & Niven, J. S. (1963). Inhibition of mantoux reaction by direct suggestion under hypnosis. British Medical Journal, 1, 1649-1652.

Blalock JE, Smith EM. the immune system: our mobile brain? Immunol Today 1985;6:115.

Blavatsky, H.P. The Secret Doctrine. Point Loma, Calif.: The Aryan Theosophical Press, 1917.

Borysenko, J. Z. (1985). Healing motives, An interview with David C. McCelland. Advances, 1 (2), 29-41.

Borysenko, Joan. 1987. Minding the Body, Minding the Mind. Reading, Mass.: Addison Wesley, 1987; 1988. New York: Bantam Books,

Bovbjerg, D, Ader, R, Cohen, N. 1982. Behaviorally conditioned suppression of a graft-versus-host response. Proc. Nat. Acad. Sci. 79: 583-585

Boyd, Doug. Roling Thunder. New York: Random House. 1974.

Bradley, L.A., Turner, R.A., Young, L.D., Agudelo, C.A., Anderson, K.O., & McDaniel, L.K. (1985). Effects of cognitive-behavioral therapy on pain behavior of rheumatoid arthritis (RA) patients: preliminary outcomes. Scandinavian Journal of Behavior Therapy, 14, 51-64.

Brener, J.M., and R.A. Kleinman. Learned control of decreases in systolic blood pressure. Nature, 226, 1063-1064, 1970.

Brennan, Barbara Ann. Hands of Light. New York: Bantam Books, 1988.

Brown, Barbara B. Recognition of aspects of consciousness through association with EEG alpha activity represented by a light signal. Psychophysiology, 1970, 6, 442-452.

Campbell, Joseph. The Hero With a Thousand Faces. Princeton: Princeton University Press, 1968.

Campbell, Joseph, with Bill Moyers. The Power of Myth. New York: Doubleday, 1988.

Cohen JJ, Crnic LS. Behavior, stress, and lymphocyte recirculation. In:Cooper EL, ed. Stress, immunity, and aging. New York: Marcel Dekker, 1984:73-80.

Cohen JJ. Stress and the human immune response: a critical review. J Burn Care Rehab 1985;6:167.

Cohen JJ. Thymus-derived lymphocytes sequestered in the bone marrow of hydrocortisone-treated mice. J Immunol 1972;108:841.

Cousins, Norman. The Healing Heart. New York: Avon Books, 1984.

Cousins, Norman. Head First, The Biology of Hope. New York: E.P.Dutton, 1989

Cupps TR, Fauci AS. Corticosteroid-mediated immunoregulation in man. Immunol Rev 1982;65:133.

Delaney, Gayle. Living Your Dreams. New York: Harper & Row, 1981.

Dennis, M. & Philippus, M.J. (1965). Hypnotic and non-hypnotic suggestion and skin response in atopic patients. The Americal Journal of Clinical Hypnosis, 7(4), 342-345.

Dillon, K.M., & Baker, K.H. (1985). Positive emotional states and enhancement of the immune system. International Journal of Psychiatry in Medicine, 15(1), 13-18.

Evans, Elida. A Psychological Study of Cancer. New York: Dodd, Mead & Co., 1926.

Evans-Wentz, W.Y. The Tibetan Book of the Dead. London: Oxford, 1927. New York, Oxford University Press, 1957.

Fadiman, James. The Council Grove Conference on altered states of consciousness. J. Humanistic Psych., 9, 135-137, 1969.

Faraday, Ann. The Dream Game. New York: Harper & Row, 1976.

Ferlic, M. Goldman, A. Kennedy, B. Group counselling in adult patients with advanced breast cancer. Cancer. 43:760, 1979

Wood, P. Milligan, I, Christ, D. Liff, D. Group counselling for cancer patients in a community hospital. Psychosomatics. 19:555, 1978

Frankl, Viktor. Man's Search for Meaning. New York: Touchstone, 1984.

Franz, Marie-Louise von, with Fraser Boa. The Way of the Dream. Toronto: Windrose Films Ltd., 1987.

Furth, Gregg. The Secret Work of Drawings: Healing Through Art. Boston: Sigo Press, 1988.

Garfield, Patricia. Creative Dreaming. New York: Simon & schuster, 1974; New York: Ballantine Books, 1976.

Gendlin, Eugene. Let Your Body Interpret Your Dreams. Wilmette, Ill.: Chiron Pub., 1986.

Good, R.A. (1981). Foreword: Interactions of the body's major networks. In R. Ader (Ed.), Psychoneuroimmunology (pp. xvii-xix). New York, NY: Academic Press.

Green, Alyce M., and E. Dale Walters. Feedback technique for deep relaxation. Psychophysiology, 6, 371-377, 1969.

Green, Alyce M., and Green, Elmer E. Biofeedback: research and therapy. In Nils Jacobson, ed., New Ways to Health. Stockholm: Natur och Kultur, 1975.

Green, Elmer, and Alyce Green. Beyond Biofeedback. New York: Dell, Delta Books, 1977.

Green, R.G., & Green, M.L. (1987). Relaxation increases salivary immunoglobin A. Psychological Reports, 61, 623-629.

Green, M.L., & Green, R.L. (1985). Relaxation modifies salivary immunoglobulin A and salivary cortisol. Unpublished manuscript, Albright College, Reading, PA.

Gruber, B.L., Hall, N.R., Hersh, S. P., & Dubois, P. (1986, August). Immune system and psychologic changes in metastatic cancer patients while using ritualized relaxation and guided imagery: A pilot study. Paper presented at the meeting of the American Psychological Association, Washington, D.C.

Hall, H., Longo, S., Dixon, R. (1981, October). Hypnosis and the immune system: The effect of hypnosis on T and B cell function. Paper presented to the Society for Clinical Experimental Hypnosis, 33rd annual meeting, Portland, Oregon.

Harrison, A.M., Fahs, D.E., Fehredbach, D., Hooper, M.C., Landis, T., Mathur, C.F., & Novotny, P.E. (1986). Immune parameters are enhanced by relaxation. Unpublished manuscript, York College, York, PA.

Hertzler, Arthur. The Horse and Buggy Doctor. New York: Harper & Row, 1938.

Hogan M, Olness K, MacDonald J: Self-hypnosis and voluntary control of brainstem auditory evoked potentials in childred. Am J Clin Hypn 1985;3:91-94

Huxley, Aldous. The Doors of Perception. New York: Harper & Row, 1970.

Ikemi, Y., & Nakagawa, S. (1962). A psychosomatic study of contagious dermatitis. Kyushu Journal of Medical Science, 13, 335-350.

Jacobs S, Ostfeld A. An epidemiological review of the mortality of bereavement. Psychosom Med 1977;39:344.

Jasnoski, M.L. & Kugler, J. (1987). Relaxation, imagery, and neuroimmunomodulation. Annals of the New York Academy of Sciences, 496, 723-730.

Jemmott JB, Borysenko JZ, Borysenko M, McClelland DC, Chapman R, Meyer D, Benson H. Academic stress, power motivation, and decrease in secretion rate of salivary secretory immunoglobin A. Lancet 1983;1:1400.

Jung, Carl G. Man and His Symbols. New York: Dell, 1968.

-----. Memories, Dreams, Reflections. Edited by Aniela Jaffe. Translated by Richard and Clara Winston. New York: Vintage, 1965.

-----. The Structure of Dynamics of the Psyche. 2nd ed. Princeton: Princeton University Press, 1968.

Justice, Blair. Who Gets Sick? Los Angeles: J.P. Tarcher, 1988. Distributed by St. Martin's Press, New York.

Kaneko, Z., & Takaishi, N. (1963). Psychosomatic studies on chronic urticaria. Folia Psychiatrica et Neurologica, 17(1), 17-24.

Keenedy, S, Kiecolt-Glaser, J, Glaser, R. Immunological consequences of acute and chronic stressors: mediating role of interpersonal relationships. Br J Med Psychol. 61:77, 1988

Kiecolt-Glaser, J.K., Glaser, R., Strain, E, Stout, J.C., Tarr, K.L., Holliday, J.E., & Speicher, C.E. Modulation of cellular immunity in medical students. Journal of Behavioral Medicine, 9:5-21, 1986.

Kiecolt-Glaser, J.K., Glaser, R., Willinger, D., Stout, J., Messick, G., Sheppard, S., Ricker, D., Romisher, S.C., Briner, W., Bonnell, G., & Donnerberg, R. (1985). Psychosocial enhancement of immmunocompetence in a geriatric population. Health Psychology, 4, 25-41.

Kiecolt-Glaser JK, Stephens RE, Lipetz PD et al: Distress and DNA repair in human lymphocytes. J Behav Med 1985;8:311-320

Kluger MJ, Oppenheim JO, Powanda MC, eds. The physiologic, metabolic, and immunologic actions of interleukin-1. New York: Alan R. Liss, 1985.

Kosslyn, Stephen M. *Image and Mind*. Cambridge, MA: Harvard University Press. 1980

Kronfol Z, Silva J, Gieden J, et al: Impaired lymphocyte function n depressive illness. Life Sci 1983;33:241-247

Kubler-Ross, Elizabeth. On Death and Dying. New York: Macmillan, 1969.

LeShan, Lawrence. How to Meditate. Boston: Little, Brown, 1974; New York: Bantam Books, 1984.

LeShan, Lawrence. You Can Fight for Your Life: Emotional Factors in the Causation of Cancer. New York: Evans, 1977.

LeShan, Lawrence, and Margenau, Henry. Einstein's Space and Van Gogh's Sky. New York. Macmillan. 1982.

Locke SE, Hurst MW, LeSeiman JM, et al: Life change stress and human natural killer cell activity, in Behavioral Immunology. New York, Praeger, 1983

Locke, Steven, and Douglas Colligan. The Healer Within. New York: Dutton, 1986; New York: New American Library, Mentor Books, 1987.

Locke, Steven, Robert Ader, Hugo Besedovsky, Nicholas Hall, George Solomon, and Tery Strom,eds. and N. Herbert Spector, consulting ed., Foundation of *Psychoneuroimmunology*, New York:Aldine, 1985.

Long, M. The Secret Science Behind Miracles. Vista, Calif.: Huna Research Publication, 1948.

Low, Abraham. *Mental Training Through Will-training*. Winnetka, Illnois: Willett Publishing Co. 1950

Mason, A.A., & Black, S. (1958). Allergic skin responses abolished under treatment of asthma and hayfever by hypnosis. Lancet, 1, 877-880.

McClelland DC, Floor E, Davidson RJ, Saron C. Stressed power motivation, sympathetic activation, immune function, and illness. J Human Stress 1980;6:11.

McClelland, D.C., (1988). The effect of motivational arousal through films on salivary immunoglobulin A. Psychology and Health, 2, 31-52.

Menninger, Karl. Love Against Hate. New York: Harcourt, Brace & Co., 1942.

Menninger, Karl, with Martin Mayman and Paul Pruyser. The Vital Balance. New York: Viking Press, 1963; Magnolia, Mass.: Peter Smith, 1963.

Menninger, Karl. Man Against Himself. New York: Harcourt, Brace & Co., 1938.

Miller, Stuart, Naomi Remen, Allen Barbour, Sara Miller, and Dale Garrell. Dimensions of Humanistic Medicine. San Francisco: Institute for the Study of Medicine, 1975.

Mindell, Arnold. Dreambody. Boston: Sigo Press, 1982.

Mindell, Arnold. Working With the Dreaming Body. London and New York: Routledge & Kegan Paul, 1985.

Norris, P, and Porter, G. I Choose Life. Walpole, New Hampshire. Stillpoint Publishing. 1987

Nouwen, Henri. Out of Solitude. Notre Dame, Ind.: Ave Maria Press, 1974.

Olness, K, Conroy M: Voluntary control of transcutaneous P02 by children: A pilot study. Int J Clin Exp Hypn 1985;33:1-5

Olness, K., Culbert, T., and Uden, D. Self-Regulation of Dalivary Immunoglobulin A by Children. Pediatrics 1989;83:66-71

Olness J: Imagery: Self-hypnosis as adjunct therapy in childhood cancer: Clinical experience with 25 patients. Am J Pediat Hematol Oncol 1981;3:313-321

Olness, K, MacDonald JT, Uden DL: Comparison of self-hypnosis and propranolol in the treatment of juvenile classic migraine. Pediatrics 1987;79:593-597

Ornstein, Robert, and David Sobel. The Healing Brain. New York: Simon & Schuster, 1987.

Oyle, Irving. The Healing Mind. New York: Pockets Books, 1975.

Peavey, B.S., Lawlis, G.F., & Goven, A. (1985). Biofeedback and Self-Regulation, 10, 33-47.

Peck, M.S., The Road Less Travelled. New York. Simon and Schuster. 1978.

Rider, M.S. & Achterberg, J. The effect of music-mediated imagery on neutrophils and lymphocytes. Submitted to Biofeedback and Self-Regulation.

Rosen, Sidney. My Voice Will Go With You: The Teaching Tales of Milton H. Erickson, M.D. New York: W.W. Norton & Co., 1982.

Rossi, Ernest L. The Psychobiology of Mind-Body Healing. New York: W.W. Norton & Co., 1986.

Rossi, Ernest L., and David Cheek. Mind-body Therapy: Methods of Ideodynamic Healing and Hypnosis. New York: W.W. Norton & Co., 1988.

Sagan, Carol. The Cosmic Connection. New York: Doubleday, 1973.

Samuels, Mike, and Nancy Samuels. Seeing With the Mind's Eye. New York: Random House, 1975.

Saroyan, William. The Human Comedy. New York: Harcourt, Brace, World, 1971.

Schleifer SJ, Keller SE, Camerino E, Thomton JC, Stein M. Suppression of lymphocyte stimulation following bereavement. JAMA 1983;250:374.

Schmale AH, Iker H. Hopelessness as a predictor of cervical cancer. Soc Sci Med 1971;5:95-100.

Schneider, J., Smith, C.W., & Whitcher, S. (1984). The relationship of mental imagery to white blood cell (neutrophil) function: Experimental studies of normal subjects. Paper presented at the 36th annual convention of the Society for Clinical and Experimental Hypnosis, San Antonio, Texas.

Schultz, Johannes. The clinical importance of "inward seeing" in autogenic training. British Journal of Medical Hypnotism, II, 26-28, 1960.

Schultz, Johannes, and Wolfgang Luthe. Autogenic Training: A Psychophysiologic Approach in Psychotherapy. New York: Grune * Stratton, 1959.

Selye, Hans. The Stress of Life. Rec. ed. New York: McGraw-Hill, 1976.

Shah, Idries. The Way of the Sufi. London: Jonathan Cape, 1968.

Shealy, C. Norman, and Arthur S. Freese. Occult Medicine Can Save Your Life. New York: Dial, 1975.

Shertzer, C.L. & Lookingbill, D.P. (1987). Effects of relaxation therapy and hypnotizability in chronic urticaria. Archives of Dermatology, 123, 913-916.

Siegel, B.S. Love, Medicine, and Miracles. New York: Harper & Row. 1986.

Siegel, B.S. Peace, love & healing: bodymind communication and the path to self-healing: an exploration. New York: Harper & Row, 1989.

Simonton, O. Carl, Stephanie Matthews-Simonton and James Creighton. Getting Well Again. Los Angeles: J.P. Tarcher, 1978; New York: Bantam Books, 1980.

Skinner, B.F. Beyond Freedom and Dignity. New York: Knopf, 1972.

Smith, G.R. (in press). Intentional psychological modulation of the immune system. In J.V. Basmajian (Ed.), Biofeedback: Principles and Practice for Clinicians (3rd ed.). Baltimore: Williams and Wilkens.

Smith, G.R. & McDaniel, S.M. (1983). Psychologically mediated effect on the delayed hypersensitivity reaction to tuberculin in humans. Psychosomatic Medicine, 45, 65-70.

Smith, G.R., McKenzie, J.M., Marmer, D.J., & Steele, R.W. (1985). Psychologic modulation of the human immune response to varicella zoster. Archives of Internal Medicine, 145, 2210-2212.

Solzhenitsyn, Aleksandr. Cancer Ward. Translated by Nicholas Bethell and David Burg. New York: Farar, Straus & Giroux, 1969; New York: Bantam Books, 1969.

Teilhard de Chardin, Pierre. The Phenomenon of Man. New York: Harper, 1959.

Thomas, Lewis. The Youngest Science. New York: Viking Press, 1983; New York: Bantam Books, 1984.

Tolstoy, Leo. The Death of Ivan Illich. Available in various editions.

Williams JM, Peterson RG, Shea PA, Schmedtje JF, Bauer DC, Felten DL. Sympathetic innervation of murine thymus and spleen: evidence for a functional link between the nervous and immune systems. Brain Res Bull 1981;6:83.

References for Aging

Ali, M. Nutritional Medicine: Principles and Practice. Bloomfield, New Jersey: Institute of Preventive Medicine. 1990

Ali, M. The Agony and Death of a Cell, in Syllabus of the American Academy of Environmental Medicine. Denver, Colorado. 1988.

Ali, M. Immunity is our Capacity to Preserve Health, in Syllabus of the American Academy of Environmental Medicine. Denver, Colorado, 1988.

Ali, M. and Fayemi, A. Pathology of Maintenance Dialysis. Springfield, Illinois. Charles Thomas Publishers,1982

Ali, M., Fayemi, A., and Braun, E., Surgical Pathology. New York. Medical Examination Publishing Company. 1978.

Ali, M., Braun, E., and Fayemi, A., Pathology. New York. Medical Examination Publishing Company. 1980

Ali, M. et al Pathology review. New York. Medical Examination Publishing Company. 1976.

Atkins, Robert. Health Revolution. Boston, Houghton Mifflin Co. 1988.

Atkins, Robert. Diet Revolution. New York: David McKay Co. 1972

Bland, J. (ed) Yearbook of Nutritional Medicine. New Canaan, C.T. Keats Publishers. 1985.

Bradford, R, Allen, H. Culbert, M. Oxidology. Los Altos, California. The Robert W. Bradford Foundation. 1985

Budwig, J. Das Fettsyndrom. Freiberg, W. Germany. Hyperion Verlag. 1959

Chen, L. H., An increase in vitamin E requirement induced by high supplementation of vitamin C in rats, Am. J. Clin. Nutr., 34 1036, 1981.

Chen, L. H., Effect of vitamin E and selenium on tissue antioxidant status of rats, J. Nutr., 103, 503, 1973.

Chen, L. H., (ed) Nutritional Aspects of Aging. Boca Raton, Florida. CRC Press, 1986.

Chow, Ch. K., Nutritional influence on cellular antioxidant defense systems, Am. J. Clin. Nutr., 32, 1066, 1979.

Clandinin, M. T. and Innis, S. M., Does mitochondrial ATP synthesis decline as a function of change in membrane environment with aging? Mech. Ageing Dev. 22, 205, 1983.

Clemens, M.J. (ed). Biochemistry of Cellular Regulation. Boca Raton, Florida. CRC Press, 1981.

Cutler, Richard G. Peroxide-producing of tissues: Inverse correlation with longevity of mammalian species. Pro. Nat. Aca. Sci. 82: 4798, 1985.

Epstein, J. and Gershon, D., Studies on ageing in nematodes. IV. The effect of antioxidants on cellular damage and life span, Mech. Ageing Dev., 1, 257, 1972.

Erasmus. U. Fats and Oils. Alive. Vancouver, Canada. 1986

Golos, N., O'Shea, J., Waickman, Francis., and Goblitz, F., Environmental Medicine. New Canaan, Connecticut, Keats Publishing, Inc. 1987.

Harman, D. and Eddy, D. E., Free radical theory of aging: effect of adding antioxidants to maternal mouse diets on the lifespan of their offspring - second experiment, Age, 1, 162, (#40), 1978.

Harman, D., Free radical theory of aging: beneficial effect of antioxidants on the lifespan of male NBZ mice: role of free radical reactions in the deterioration of the immune system with age and in the pathogenesis of systemic lupus erythematosus, Age, 3, 64, 1980.

Harman, D., Free radical theory of aging: consequences of mitochondrial aging, Age, 6, 86, 1983.

Harman, D., Free radical theory of aging: effect of free radical inhibitors on the mortality rate of male LAF1 mice, J. Gerontal., 23, 476, 1968.

Harman, D., Free radical theory of aging: origin of life, evolution and aging, Age, 3, 100, 1980.

Harman, D., Prolongation of the normal lifespan by radiation protection chemicals, J. Gerontal., 12, 257, 1957.

Hegner, D., Age-dependence of molecular and functional changes in biological membrane properties, Mech. Ageing Dev., 14, 101, 1980.

Jensen, Bernard and Anderson, Mark., Empty Harvest. Garden City Park, New York. Avery Publishing Group. 1990

Jones, E. and Hughes, R. E., Quercetin, flavonoids and the lifespan of mice, Exp. Gerontal., 17, 213, 1982.

Kahn-Thomas, M. and Enesco, H. E., Relation between growth rate and lifespan in alpha-tocopherol cultured Turbatrix acet, Age, 5, 46, 1982.

Kormendy, Ch. G. and Bender, A. D., Chemical interference with aging, Gerontologia, 17, 52, 1971.

Ledvina, M. and Hodanova, M., The effect of simultaneous administration of tocopherol and sunflower oil on the life span of female mice, Exp. Gerontal., 15, 67, 1980.

Levine, S. and Kidd, P. Antioxidant Adaptation. San Leandro, CA. Allergy research Group, 1985.

Miquel, J., Binnard, R., and Fleming, J. E., Role of metabolic rate and

DNA repair in Drosophila aging: implications for the mitochondrial mutation theory of aging, Exp. Gerontal., 18, 167, 1983.

Miquel, J. and Economos, A. C., Factorable effects of the antioxidants sodium and magnesium thiazolidine carboxylate on the vitality and lifespan of Drosophila and mice, Exp. Gerontal., 14, 279, 1979.

Miquel, J., Fleming, J., and Economos, A. C., Antioxidants, metabolic rate and aging in Drosophila, Arch. Gerontal. Geriatr., 1, 159, 1982.

Moment, G.B.,(ed) Nutritional Approaches to Aging Research, Boca Raton, Florida, CRC Press, 1982.

National Research council. Recommended daily allowances. Washington.DC: National Academy Press. 1989.

Oeriu, S. and Vochitu, E., The effects of the administration of compounds which contain -SH groups on the survival rate of mice, rats and guinea pigs, J. Gerontal., 20, 417, 1965.

Patel, V., Miquel, J., Sharma, H. M., and Johnson, J. E., Hypocholesterolemic action of the antioxidants tocopherol p-chlorophenoxyacetate and magnesium thiazolidine carboxylate, Age, 2, 33, 1979.

Randolph, Theron. Environmental Medicine. Fort Collins, Colorado. Clinical Ecology Publications, Inc. 1987.

Randolph, Theron.Human Ecology and Susceptibility to the Chemical Environment. Springfield. Illinois. Charles C. Thomas, 1962.

Rapp, Doris. The Impossible Child. Buffalo: Practical Allergy Research Foundation. 1986.

Reddy, B.S., and Cohen, L.A. Diet, Nutrition, and Cancer. Boca Raton, Florida. CRC Press, 1986

Richie, J. P., Mills, B. J., and Lang, C. A., Magnesium thiazolidine-4-carboxylic acid increases both glutathione levels and longevity, Gerontologist, 23, 67, 1983.

Rinkel, H., Randolph, T,. and Zeller, M. Food Allergy. Springfield, Illinois: Charles C. Thomas. 1951

Rogers, Sherry. Toxic or Tired. Syracuse, New York. Prestige Publishing. 1990.

Rohlfing, D., Oparin, A, Molecular evolution: Prebiological and Biological, New York. Planum Press, 1972

Rousseau, David., Rea, W.J., Enright, Jean. Your Home, Your Health, and Well-Being. Vancouver, B.C. Hartley and Marks, Ltd. 1987.

Ruddle, D. L., Yengoyan, L. S., Fleming, J. E., and Miquel, J., Effects of structurally diverse antioxidants on the lifespan of Drosophila, Gerontologist, 23, 24A, 1983.

Tolmasoff, Julie., Ono, Tetsuya., Cutler, Richard., Superoxide Dismutase: Correlation with life-span and specific metabolic rate in primate species. Pro. Nat. Aca. Sci. 77:2777, 1980.

Walford, R.L. Maximum Life Span. New York. W.W. Norton & Co. 1983.

Weber, J. U., Fleming, J. F., and Miquel, J., Thiazolidine-4-carboxylic acid, a physiologic sulfhydryl antioxidant with potential value in geriatric medicine, Arch. Gerontal. Geriatr., 1, 299, 1982.

*That which is true is not necessarily
that which is accepted.*

Robert C. Atkins, M.D.

About the author

When asked if a *Sufi of molecular medicine* best describes him, Dr. Ali responded, "I don't know if I deserve that title but that does describe my work."

In the section on *Ten Lessons Learned From Patients*, Dr. Ali describes his journeys through the worlds of human organs, cells, and molecules. He writes about his sojourns in the worlds of the molecules of the physiology of fitness, of the pharmacology of nutrients, of the chemistry of environments, of the immunology of allergy, of the pathology of autoimmune dysfunctions, and of the biology of self-regulation. He speaks about his travels through the worlds of teachers and pupils, of controversy and conflict, of human suffering and of the crises of life and death. He writes,

> *"I was being prepared, it seems. Prepared for what? For self-regulation!! This thought never crossed my mind."*

Dr. Ali is a fellow of the Royal College of Surgeons of England, a diplomate of the American Board of Anatomic Pathology, and a diplomate of the American Board of Clinical

Pathology. He is a member of the teaching faculty of the American Academy of Environmental Medicine.

Dr. Ali attended King Edward Medical College in Lahore, Pakistan. He received his surgical training in Mayo Hospital, Lahore, Princess Margaret Hospital, Swindon, England, Swansea Hospital, Swansea, Wales, and Jersey City Medical Center in Jersey City, New Jersey. He received his training in surgical and clinical pathology at Holy Name Hospital, Teaneck, New Jersey and at Columbia Presbyterian Hospital in New York City.

Since 1974, Dr. Ali has served as Director of Pathology, Immunology and Laboratories at Holy Name Hospital, Teaneck, New Jersey. In 1985 and 1986, he was elected to serve two terms as the President of the Medical Staff of Holy Name. He is an Associate Professor of Pathology (adj) at the College of Physicians and Surgeons of Columbia University in New York.

Dr. Ali is the author or co-author of 11 books on various subjects in pathology, immunology and allergy. He has published over 75 scientific papers in national and international journals.

Of his various interests, he is most at ease when behind his microscope and when teaching his patients self-regulation and healing.

Dr. Ali lives in Teaneck, New Jersey with his wife, Talat. Their three children, Sarah, Omar and Amir attend schools at Cornell University, Boston College and Lehigh University, respectively.